To my respected friend and colleague
in appreciation and recognition of his ma...
field of dental materials

Thys Vrijhoef.

M. M. A. Vrijhoef / A. G. Vermeersch / A. J. Spanauf

# Dental Amalgam

# Dental Amalgam

*Matthijs M. A. Vrijhoef*
University of Nijmegen

*Albert G. Vermeersch*
University of Louvain

*Adam J. Spanauf*
University of Nijmegen

Quintessence Publishing Co., Inc. 1980
Chicago, Berlin, Rio de Janeiro and Tokyo

Lithography: Industrie- und Presseklischee, Berlin
Composition: Kupijai & Prochnow, Berlin
Printing: Universal Printing Co., St. Louis
Binding: Becktold Co., St. Louis
Printed in U.S.A.

ISBN 0-931386-16-0

"Dental alloys are manufactured for us. Amalgam we make for ourselves, and the strength and the stability of the hardened amalgam and the merit of the filling are only as good as the care and the skill the dentist puts into it".

William E. Harper, J. Am. Dent. Assoc. **13,** 119–125, 1926.

# Contents

# 1. General Introduction

## 1.1. Motivation for the Book

The authors of the present monograph about dental amalgam are fully aware of the difficulty of their task. On the one hand, it is desirable to make a textbook for the dental student, who first encounters the problems related to this restorative material on a rather theoretical basis. On the other hand dental practitioners, already familiar with the peculiarities of amalgam restorations, feel the necessity for a book which makes it clear that the new developments as to the material and new theoretical progress can be related directly to their practice situation. The general practitioner has more interest in the practical repercussions of new developments than in the theoretical background.

The dental student will learn to know all the basic principles and theories concerning dental amalgam. As soon as he is working with dental amalgam he will experience it to be probably the most difficult, extremely exacting, unexpectedly capricious, but also the most docile material as long as perfection is the main objective and an intelligent manipulation is applied. As stated by Aesop the tongue represents the best and the worst amongst things; amalgam restorations might be the most noble restorations but also the worst "ignoble fillings".

Making an amalgam restoration might be considered to be a chain process. Because the strength of a chain depends upon its weakest link, the misjudgment of its properties or the smallest neglect as to its manipulation might have unfavourable repercussions with regard to the restoration and even result in its total failure. We hope that this book will help the student have a good start and will enable him to straighten out certain problems.

As it has been pointed out, this book is also intended for the general practitioner who both has the impression already to know the material and who uses it frequently. We would like to ask them immediately: "Are you satisfied with the material?" Only those amongst them who never evaluate their own work critically will be inclined to say "it works jolly well". However, we sincerely hope the majority will answer negatively. They experience from time to time dimensional instability of the restoration, sometimes come across a bulk fracture, observe unacceptable corrosion and marginal deterioration of the restoration, find fracture of the enamel margins, detect discoloration of the adjacent hard tissue or recurrent caries. They will also have problems with reading advertisements with regard to new products, not knowing how to interpret data as to the strength, creep or other properties, being completely

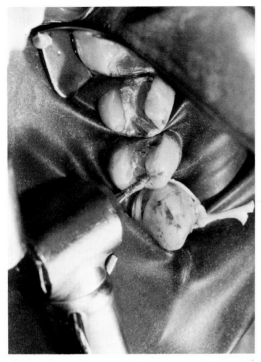

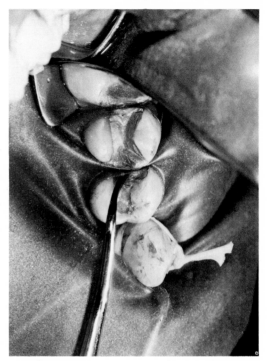

Fig. 1 An amalgam cavity prepared with a small diamond stone.

Fig. 2 The cervical margin of a class II amalgam preparation finished with a gingival margin trimmer.

confused about the clinical repercussions of these figures.

These dental practitioners will be aware of the fact that amalgam certainly has its imperfections rather than being an ideal restorative material. They will be fully aware of the situation that many an amalgam restoration failure is closely related to a faulty manipulation of the material as they are conscious of the golden rule that no amalgam restoration is better than the operator who made it. This book will enable them to distinguish between the different iatrogenic factors determining success and failure of an amalgam restoration in the oral environment such as cavity preparation, special precautions to keep the field of operation dry, the importance of the alloy choice, an ideal dosage of alloy and mercury, the mode of mixing, condensation, carving and polishing. Furthermore, the practice may show that some properties are more relevant than others.

We hope that, after turning to the last page of this book, the dental student has acquired the necessary knowledge for the correct use of modern amalgam alloys. As to the dental practitioners we hope that they have gained some insight with respect to recent developments in the field of dental amalgam and strengthened their clinical view, thereby

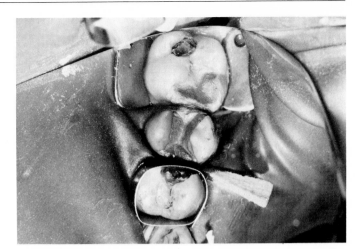

Fig. 3 A class II amalgam cavity with individual matrix band and wedge; ready to be restored.

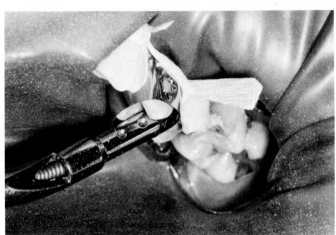

Fig. 4 Application of amalgam into a prepared cavity with an amalgam carrier.

contributing to a better recognition of the casualties related to amalgam restorations and a more sophisticated problem solving.

## 1.2. Summary of the Chapters

Chapter 2 summarizes the compositon and microstructure of amalgam alloys and their corresponding amalgams.

Amalgam restorations have been used in dentistry for over 150 years. At the turn of the nineteenth century G. V. Black recommended "an improved" lathe cut alloy containing 68% silver with smaller quantities of tin, copper and zinc. This formula has been the basis for our present conventional composition alloys. Apart from some modifications, this alloy has been used for 75 years approximately. Only in the sixties spherical alloys and materials with a different composition were introduced.

13

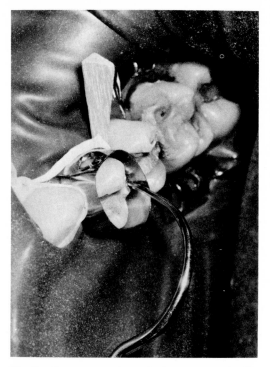

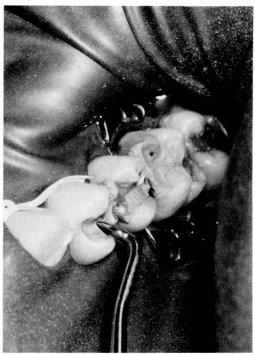

Fig. 5 Excess amalgam being removed with a sickle shaped probe before taking off the matrix band in order not to fracture the marginal ridge.

Fig. 6 Carving instrument being used to bring and refine the occlusal anatomy in the amalgam restoration.

Furthermore, these changes have been accompanied by a reduction of the particle size. The microstructural parameters of both the amalgam alloy and the amalgam received a lot of attention before the second world war. However, only very recently, it became very clear that properties of the amalgam alloy such as its reactivity with mercury and the hardening mechanism as well as the properties of the amalgam, and thereby the functioning of the corresponding restorations under oral conditions depend upon these factors. Especially after the introduction of the spherical and dispersant type alloys an avalanche of new information became available. Chapter 2 will cover this data and trace the progress made during the last 75 years.

Chapter 3 is dealing with the pertinence of the properties of amalgam as to the functioning of amalgam restorations. Furthermore, attention is given to the fact whether alloy choice and manipulation of the amalgam significantly influence the clinical quality and stability of amalgam restorations. For instance it is pointed out that strength after setting is a relevant property. However, as to the significance of materials choice and handling it will be clarified that these

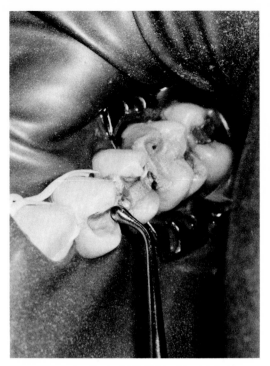

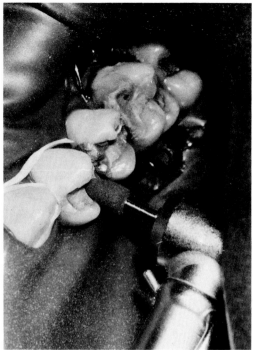

Fig. 7 All accessible places of the amalgam restoration are burnished with an egg shaped ball burnishing instrument.

Fig. 8 The inital finishing of an amalgam restoration with an abrasive point.

factors are not (any more) significant as long as the dental practitioner adheres to generally accepted rules as to the cavity preparation and the amalgam manipulation. The knowledge acquired in this chapter not only can be applied in relation to materials choice and manipulation versus the ultimate life time of amalgam restorations, but it is also useful for reading advertisements produced by the manufacturers. For example, from section 3.3.2.2. it will become clear that a manufacturer claiming a better amalgam because the diametral tensile strength after hardening is 56 MN/m², should be considered to preach qualified nonsense. Repercussions of properties of amalgam as to the cavity design and morphology of the restoration will be dealt with.

As far as the manipulation is concerned, attention will be paid to the borderland between "accepted clinical technique" and "bad practice".

In chapter 4 it is dealt with the relation between on the one hand composition and microstructure of the amalgam (alloy) and on the other hand the properties of the amalgam. The influence exerted by the dental team upon composition and microstructure will be described so as to make it feasible to

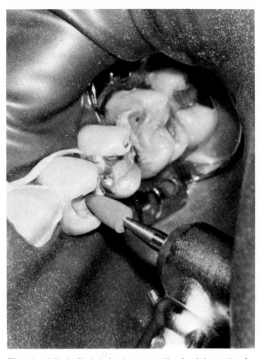 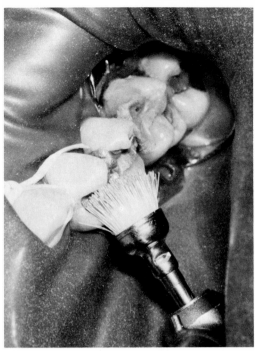

Fig. 9   High finish being applied with a shofu rubber point.

Fig. 10   The high polish being applied with a bristle and a fluoride containing pumice.

predict the influence of manipulation upon properties and thereby the functioning of an amalgam restoration under oral conditions.

Chapter 5 is a practical elaboration of chapter 4. It gives some practical guidelines as to alloy choice, proportioning of alloy and mercury, trituration, condensation, carving and polishing.

## 1.3. Placing an Amalgam Restoration

It is not within the scope of this book to deal with all aspects related to cavity preparation and the manipulation of the amalgam. However, in order to make it possible to read this book, some nomenclature and basic knowledge as to the restorative procedure is necessary. This section supplies this need for the dental freshman.

A dental amalgam is obtained by reaction of mercury and a metal powder (dental amalgam alloy). After proportioning the dental amalgam alloy and the mercury these components are mixed. This mixing process is generally defined as trituration. After trituration has been completed a plastic mass is obtained which is condensed (i. e. packed) into the prepared cavity by means of suitable packing instruments. Next, the restoration is carved to the correct

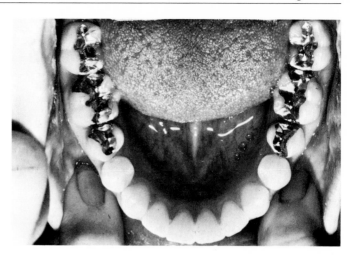

Fig. 11   A full lower arch restored with dental amalgam.

anatomical contours. After complete setting of the amalgam the restoration is polished. A photographic overview of the restorative treatment is given in the figures of this chapter. For the respective aspects of amalgam manipulation it is referred to chapter 5.

## 1.4. Acknowledgments

The authors wish to express their gratitude and indebtness to the following people who contributed so much to help make this first edition a complete textbook. Special gratitude must be acknowledged to Mr. *F. L. Lourens* and Mrs. *A. F. M. Leijdekkers-Govers* for their contribution to many experiments. To Prof. Dr. *F. C. M. Driessens* for reading parts of the manuscript. Thanks are due to Mrs. *M. A. G. Bosmans-Friedrichs* for performing the difficult task of typing the manuscript, and Dr. *B. M. Spanauf-Bester* for correcting the language. Acknowledgment is also due to Mr. *J. L. M. v. d. Kamp* and Mr. *H. A. W. Bongaarts* from the photographic department and Mr. *H. C. M. Reckers* and Mr. *H. M. Berris* from the graphic department. The authors wish to thank Mr. *M. A. O. v. Groningen* for his valuable advice and help. Last but not least we would like to thank our librarian Mr. *L. J. H. Hofman*.

# 2. Composition and Microstructure of Amalgam Alloys and Their Amalgams

## 2.1. Introduction

In general, composition and microstructure of a material are extremely important. These two parameters usually determine the properties, and therefore also the behavior under certain conditions. In case of dental amalgam, already in the stage of manipulation of the amalgam mass, the dentist is implicitly confronted with features such as the chemical composition and (micro) structure. These parameters determine the plasticity of the amalgam mass, the working time as well as the setting time. After hardening, compositional and microstructural parameters determine whether attacks from the aggressive oral environment will be successful. If these harmful effects are successful the initial quality of the restoration deteriorates and the functioning of the restoration becomes more and more unsatisfactory till the point of complete failure is reached leading to the replacement of the old restoration by a new one.

In this chapter an enumeration will be presented as to the most important aspects with respect to the chemical composition and microstructure of commercially available dental amalgam alloys and their corresponding amalgams. The relation of composition and microstructure with properties, and thereby with the functioning of the restoration in the oral cavity, as well as with all means available to the general practitioner to influence them, will be dealt with at greater length in chapter 4 and 5.

## 2.2. Composition of the Amalgam Alloy and Amalgam

Not so long ago, the composition of the commercially available amalgam alloys generally fell within the limits required by the former ADA specification no. 1; their composition essentially being the same as the most successful alloys investigated by *G. V. Black* (1895, 1896). A more or less representative chemical composition of a dental amalgam alloy within the required specification limits might be: silver (Ag)—70 wt.%, tin (Sn)—26 wt% and copper (Cu)—4 wt.% Sometimes, up to 2 wt.% zinc (Zn) is added, whereas, especially in Europe, up to 3 wt.% mercury (Hg) is present as a component of some alloys. Recently, alloys with a substantial different composition have been introduced on the market. All of them are characterized by a higher copper content. This trend of incorporating more copper in the amalgam alloy can be assessed from table 1. The chemical composition of several traditional and high copper amalgam alloys are given in table 2.

*Black* (1895, 1896) already investigated alloys containing components such as bismuth (Bi), gold (Au), platinum (Pt),

Table 1
Chemical composition range of commercial amalgam alloys in comparison with the primary ADA specification limits.

| Element | ADA limits* | Schoen-makers (1967) | ADA (1968) | Vrijhoef et al. (1975) | (1976) | (1977) |
|---------|-------------|----------------------|------------|------------------------|--------|--------|
| Silver  | ≧ 65 | 66.0–70.7 | 66.7–74.5 | 66.4–72.6 | 58.7–72.7 | 41.2–72.7 |
| Tin     | ≦ 29 | 25.3–26.8 | 25.3–27.0 | 24.8–28.9 | 17.7–29.4 | 15.1–30.2 |
| Copper  | ≦  6 | 2.4– 5.4  | 0.0– 6.0  | 1.1– 5.4  | 1.4–13.0  | 1.4–28.3  |
| Zinc    | ≦  2 | 0.0– 1.9  | 0.0– 1.9  | 0.0– 1.9  | 0.0– 1.8  | 0.0– 1.8  |
| Mercury | ≦  3 | 0.0– 2.7  | not given | 0.0– 3.0  | 0.0– 3.2  | 0.0– 3.2  |

* Recently, after the introduction of the high copper alloys, wider limits have been accepted.

palladium (Pd), aluminium (Al) and cadmium (Cd). Recently, alloys containing gold (*Johnson* et al., 1973), nickel (Ni) (*Vaidyanathan & Greener,* 1976), manganese (Mn) (*Waterstrat, Rupp & Manuszewski,* 1976) and indium (In) (*Shofu,* 1976) have been (re) considered. *Tobler, Rostocker & Massler* (1974) proposed $AgCd_3$ and Cd–10 wt.% Ni amalgam alloys. At present, none of them but one (Indiloy of the Shofu Dental Corporation, containing In) is available as a commercial alloy. Once the amalgam is formed, it contains between 40 and 55 wt.% mercury approximately. The average mercury content as well as the distribution of mercury over the restoration depends upon both the initial mercury content during trituration and the condensation technique.

In general, amalgams made from spherical alloys contain less mercury than those ones made from lathe cut alloys (see chapter 5).

## 2.3. Particle Form and Size of the Amalgam Alloy

Conventional composition alloys are delivered either as fillings or as spherical particles. The fillings are cut from an ingot. Milling and sifting give the ultimate particle size, particle size distribution, as well as the ultimate form of the alloy particles. As might be judged from the two examples given in fig. 12 the actual particle form and size of the lathe cut type alloys may vary substantially. The alloy powder of a commercial alloy is a blend of different particles sizes. Caul, Barton & Manuszewski (1968) reported the particles of a particular alloy to vary considerably. Some of the finest particles may be even as small as a few microns. The length of the large particles in commercial lathe cut alloys ranged from 60 to 320 μm, the width from 10 to 70 μm and the thickness from 10 to 35 μm. Recently, the particle size of the commercial alloys has become smaller.

Some other conventional composition alloys are delivered as so-called spheri-

Table 2
Chemical composition and alloy type of some commercial amalgam alloys.

| Amalgam alloy | Alloy£ type | Chemical composition (wt. %) | | | | | |
|---|---|---|---|---|---|---|---|
| | | Ag | Sn | Cu | Zn | Hg | Other |
| Cavex SF | 2 | 72.7 | 25.8 | 1.5 | 0.0 | 0.0 | – |
| Cavex SF | 2 | 72.4 | 25.6 | 1.5 | 0.3 | 0.0 | – |
| New True Dentalloy | 1 | 70.9 | 25.8 | 2.4 | 1.0 | 0.0 | – |
| Revalloy | 1 | 70.5 | 25.8 | 2.8 | 1.1 | 0.0 | – |
| Cavex 68 | 1 | 68.2 | 26.7 | 4.9 | 0.0 | 0.0 | – |
| Cavex | 1 | 66.3 | 26.3 | 5.2 | 1.8 | 0.0 | – |
| Novalgaam | 1 | 70.4 | 24.6 | 1.4 | 0.4 | 3.2 | – |
| Splitter 67 | 1 | 66.3 | 29.4 | 2.9 | 1.0 | 0.0 | – |
| Ultra Alloy | 1 | 71.6 | 25.7 | 2.5 | 0.0 | 0.0 | – |
| Ultra Alloy | 1 | 71.9 | 25.6 | 1.5 | 1.1 | 0.0 | – |
| Solila | 1 | 70.5 | 25.4 | 2.7 | 0.0 | 1.4 | – |
| Shofu | 2 | 69.2 | 28.0 | 3.0 | 0.0 | 0.0 | – |
| Agestan 68 | 1 | 66.4 | 26.2 | 4.1 | 1.1 | 2.2 | – |
| Standalloy | 1 | 67.3 | 26.0 | 5.1 | 0.0 | 1.6 | – |
| Standalloy F | 1 | 70.6 | 25.4 | 2.8 | 0.0 | 1.2 | – |
| Katalloy | 1 | 70.2 | 25.2 | 2.9 | 0.0 | 1.7 | – |
| Shofu | 2 | 68.8 | 27.8 | 2.9 | 0.3 | 0.0 | – |
| Dentoria | 1 | 65.7 | 27.8 | 4.4 | 1.5 | 0.0 | Tin Fluoride 1 |
| Dispersalloy | 3 | 69.7 | 17.7 | 11.9 | 0.9 | 0.0 | – |
| Luxalloy | 3 | 69.3 | 19.0 | 11.2 | 0.0 | 0.0 | – |
| Cupralloy | 3 | 62.1 | 15.1 | 22.7 | 0.0 | 0.0 | – |
| Tytin | 4 | 59.4 | 27.8 | 13.0 | 0.0 | 0.0 | – |
| Micro II | 3 | 70.0 | 21.0 | 8.6 | 0.3 | 0.0 | – |
| Optalloy II | 3 | 69.9 | 21.6 | 8.1 | 0.2 | 0.0 | – |
| Indiloy | 4 | 60.6 | 24.0 | 12.1 | 0.0 | 0.0 | In: 3.4 |
| Aristalloy CR | 4 | 58.7 | 28.4 | 12.9 | 0.0 | 0.0 | – |
| Sybraloy | 4 | 41.2 | 30.2 | 28.3 | 0.0 | 0.0 | – |
| Amalcap non-$\gamma_2$* | 3 | 70.2 | 19.0 | 10.9 | 0.0 | 0.0 | – |

£ 1 : conventional composition; lathe cut
 2 : conventional composition; spherical
 3 : high copper; admixture
 4 : high copper; all-in-one

 * identical to Luxalloy

cal alloys (see fig. 12). Generally, these alloys are produced by means of an atomizing process. The alloy, formed in this manner, occurs when a spray of tiny alloy drops is allowed to solidify in a gaseous or liquid environment. Although all alloys manufactured in such a way are referred to as spherical alloys, their form is not always spherical. The particles of some spherical alloys are more like irregular grown potatoes than spheres. Generally, the particle

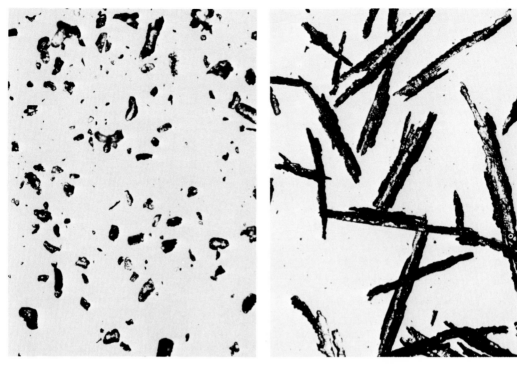

Fig. 12  Particle size and form of commercial dental amalgam alloys.

Fig. 12 a  Fine (lathe) cut, 110 x                Fig. 12 b  Course (lathe) cut, 55 x

size of the larger particles in a spherical alloy powder is 40 µm or less. A blend of spherical and lathe cut amalgam alloy is available as well.

The first commercially available high copper alloy, under the trade name Dispersalloy *(Johnson & Johnson),* was described by *Innes & Youdelis* (1963). This alloy powder is an admixture of two different powders. One part of the powder has the filing form and is of a conventional composition. The other alloy particles are spherical with an approximate composition of 72 wt.% silver and 28 wt.% copper. This composition resembles the eutectic composition of the silver-copper system approximately. An example of an admix-ture type of high copper alloy is given in fig. 12. The particle size of the lathe cut particles in this type of alloy is within the normal range. The size of the spherical eutectic particles is of the order of 10 µm or less. Subsequent and similar developments vary on this theme by changing either the chemical composition of the two alloy powders or their ratio of mixing. One system which is available, is an admixture of a conventional composition spherical alloy with a spherical silver-copper-tin alloy. Although not available on the (European) market, an amalgam alloy has been used in the U.S.A. which is an admixture of a conventional amalgam alloy and a copper amalgam (see e. g.

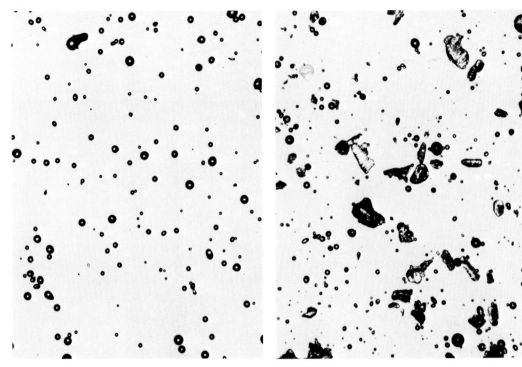

Fig. 12 c   Spherical alloy, 110 x

Fig. 12 d   High copper alloy of the admixture type. The tiny spheres are the eutectic particles, 110 x

*Marshall, Finkelstein & Greener,* 1975). In earlier days some dental practitioners used this method to produce a special amalgam alloy at the chair-side.

*Asgar* (1974) developed an all-in-one system. In this alloy all components are melted together. Up to now, these alloy particles have the spherical form. The particle size is within the range of the traditional spherical alloy particles.

Information as to the type of alloy of both some commercially available high copper alloys and several conventional composition alloys is given in table 2.

## 2.4. Phase Composition of the Amalgam Alloy

The present text books on amalgam describe the phase composition of the dental amalgam alloy on the basis of the silver-tin constitutional diagram (see fig. 13). From this diagram it is possible to deduce which phases are present under equilibrium conditions at a certain composition and temperature. For instance, in case of thermodynamic equilibrium, an alloy with 74 wt.% silver and 26 wt.% tin contains at room temperature both the $\beta$ and $\gamma$ phase. Here, the $\beta$ phase is a solid solution of tin (19.5 wt.%) in silver, whereas the $\gamma$ phase might be described approximately by the formula $Ag_3Sn$.

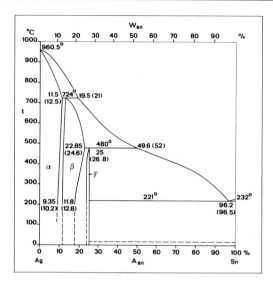

Fig. 13 Equilibrium diagram of the Ag-Sn system.

Because of the presence of copper in most amalgam alloys, the equilibrium phase composition should be described on the basis of the ternary silver-copper-tin diagram. From this diagram it is easy to conclude that, for the current commercial alloys, the $Cu_3Sn$ and $Cu_6Sn_5$ phases might be present as well (*Jensen*, 1972). No systematic research is available as to the influence of zinc and mercury upon the phase composition of the dental amalgam alloy either. However, the most serious objection against the deduction of the phase composition of the dental amalgam alloy from the silver-(copper)-tin constitutional diagram is the assumption of thermodynamic equilibrium. That such a procedure is not allowed can be made clear on the basis of the manufacturing procedures.

First step in the manufacturing process of a conventional composition lathe cut alloy is melting together the constituents. The cast ingot is given a homogenization heat treatment at 300—400°C approximately. Following this heat treatment, the ingot is reduced to filings. Then the lathe cut particles are further reduced by ball-milling. Then an ageing treatment is applied at a temperature between 100 and 150°C in order to reduce internal stresses. Times of the different heat treatments vary greatly from manufacturer to manufacturer. Several alloys supplied on the dental market are definitely not in thermodynamic equilibrium (*Jensen*, 1972; *Vrijhoef & Jensen*, 1977), demonstrating that times and temperatures in the production cycle were not appropriate to attain thermodynamic equilibrium. In the case of a spherical alloy the only usual heat treatment given is the ageing treatment at 100—150°C. This heat treatment is not sufficient to assure thermodynamic equilibrium. The influence of the homogenization treatment upon the phase composition as well as the distribution of the phases of a dental amalgam alloy is illustrated in fig. 14. In this figure an example of the microstructure of a particle of a commercial amalgam alloy powder is given as well.

In view of thermodynamics, it is obvious that no state of equilibrium can be reached in case of a high copper alloy which is an admixture of two different alloy powders. It must be stressed here that it is doubtful whether a state of thermodynamic equilibrium of the dental amalgams alloy is really a prerequisite for a good amalgam (see e. g. *Vrijhoef, Gubbels & Driessens,* 1975). The relatively good behaviour of some high copper amalgams of the admixture type as well as of some amalgams from spherical alloys underline this point of view (see chapter 3). The variability of the phase composition of some conventional composition amalgam alloys can be assessed from table 3.

Table 3
Phase composition of 21 commercial conventional composition dental amalgam alloys (Vrijhoef & Jensen, 1977).

| Phase composition* | Number of alloys |
| --- | --- |
| $\gamma + \varepsilon$ | 5 |
| $\gamma + \varepsilon + \eta'$ | 3 |
| $\gamma + \eta' + Sn$ | 3 |
| $\gamma + \beta + \varepsilon + \eta'$ | 3 |
| $\gamma + \beta + \varepsilon + \beta_1$ | 2 |
| $\gamma + \varepsilon + \eta'$ | 1 |
| $\gamma + \eta' + \beta_1$ | 1 |
| $\gamma + \beta + \eta' + Sn$ | 1 |
| $\gamma + \eta' + \beta_1 + \gamma_1$ | 1 |
| $\gamma + \varepsilon + \beta_1 + \gamma_1$ | 1 |

* $\beta$: Ag $-$ Sn ($\cong$ 20 wt. %)
 $\gamma$: $Ag_3Sn$
 $\beta_1$: Ag $-$ Hg ($\cong$ 60 wt. %)
 $\gamma_1$: Ag $-$ Hg ($\cong$ 70 wt. %)
 $\varepsilon$: $Cu_3Sn$
 $\eta'$: $Cu_6Sn_5$

## 2.5. Phase Composition of the Amalgam

Traditionally, both the amalgamation reaction of the alloy with mercury and the metallography of a conventional composition dental amalgam after setting are described on the basis of a reaction of $Ag_3Sn$ ($\gamma$) with mercury, i.e. without taking into account copper and/or zinc. During hardening, new reaction products with mercury are formed at the cost of the original alloy particles. The main reaction products formed are the $\gamma_1$ (Ag-Hg) and $\gamma_2$ (Sn-Hg) phase. This amalgamation reaction can be symbolized as follows

$$\gamma + Hg \rightarrow \gamma_1 + \gamma_2 + \gamma \text{ (remnant)}.$$

The $\gamma_1$ phase probably is the first phase formed during setting, nucleating homogeneously from the liquid mercury (Okabe, Hochman & Sims, 1975; Okabe et al., 1977a). This might be explained by the fact that silver dissolves more quickly in mercury than tin does, so that mercury gets saturated with silver before tin gets (Mitchell, Okabe & Fairhurst, 1977). At least, in some amalgams the $\gamma_2$ phase nucleates heterogeneously on the amalgam alloy particles rather than homogeneously from the mercury (Reynolds, Wawner & Wilsdorf, 1975). Although the dissolution-precipitation process probably is rate controlling in most commercially available traditional amalgams, mass transport of mercury into the alloy particles might contribute to the formation of new phases equally (Aldinger, Schuler & Petzow, 1976). After completion of the reaction, the remnants of the high melting silver-tin particles are embedded in a matrix of reaction products with mercury. In most conventional composition amalgams

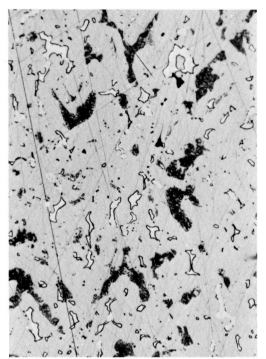 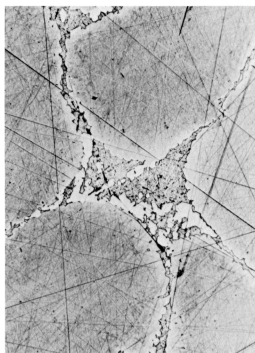

Fig. 14 Microstructure of conventional composition amalgam alloys.

Fig. 14a Ingot as cast (By permission of Quintessence International).

Fig. 14b Ingot after homogenization heat treatment (By permission of Quintessence International).

both the $\gamma_1$ and $\gamma_2$ phases form a continuous network. Probably a minor amount of amalgams shows up a $\gamma_1$ matrix in which the $\gamma_2$ phase is dispersed (see fig. 15). The distribution of the $\gamma_2$ phase is most important as to the corrosion resistance of the amalgam.

Since the early days of dental research, several suggestions have been made for the exact formula of the $\gamma_1$ and $\gamma_2$ phase on the basis of the silver-mercury and tin-mercury system. For the $\gamma_1$ phase formula have been proposed such as $Ag_4Hg_5$, $Ag_3Hg_4$, $Ag_2Hg_3$, $Ag_{11}Hg_{15}$ and $Ag_5Hg_8$ (for a review see Vrijhoef, 1973). Up to now most text books use either $Ag_2Hg_3$ or $Ag_3Hg_4$. The suggestions for the $\gamma_2$ phase vary from $Sn_7Hg$ to $Sn_8Hg$ (Vrijhoef, 1973). The controversy about the actual formula of the $\gamma_1$ and $\gamma_2$ phases was challenged by Johnson (1971) who showed the $\gamma_1$ phase to contain some tin. His findings have been subsequently confirmed by several investigators. It was shown that some copper and zinc might be present as well (Jensen et al., 1975; Mahler, Adey & Van Eysden, 1975). Apparently, the $\gamma_2$ phase contains none or only a minute amount of other components. At present, no systematic information is available as to the composition of the phases of the different commercial amalgams.

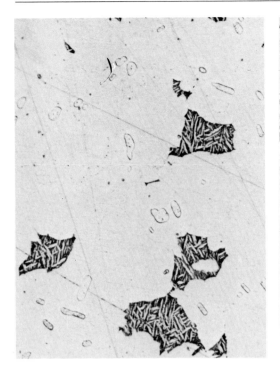

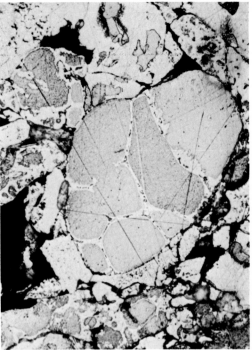

Fig. 14c Ingot after homogenization showing remnants of the Widmanstätten structure, i. e. mixture of $\gamma$ and $\beta$ phase, as well as $Cu_3Sn$ particles (Courtesy of Ing. J. C. Winkelman).

Fig. 14d Particles of a commercial alloy powder (Courtesy of Ing. J. C. Winkelman).

Although the phase composition of a freshly set dental amalgam can be described fairly well by means of the presence of $\gamma_1$ and $\gamma_2$ phases, there are some complications in that sense that some other phases are formed as well. Ageing of the amalgams reveals the $\beta_1$ (Ag-Hg-Sn) phase to be formed (see fig. 16).

The $Cu_6Sn_5$ can be formed by reaction of copper, dissolved in the $\gamma$ or $\beta$ phase, with tin ($6Cu + 5Sn \rightarrow Cu_6Sn_5$) as well as by combination of $Cu_3Sn$ with tin ($2Cu_3Sn + 3Sn \rightarrow Cu_6Sn_5$) (Vrijhoef & Driessens, 1973). Research data have shown the amalgam to be in a state of non-equilibrium for a period of time which may be in the order of one year (Vrijhoef & Driessens, 1974). Theoretical computations justify the experimental data showing initially the amalgam is not in a state of equilibrium (Reynolds & Barker, 1975).

From this section so far, it is obvious that a general description of the setting reaction of dental amalgam is very complex. Because the initial phase composition of the alloys varies substantially, it is acceptable that different reaction mechanisms hold true for the distinct types. At this time, almost no information is available as to the reactivity with mercury of the different phases present in commercial amalgam alloys.

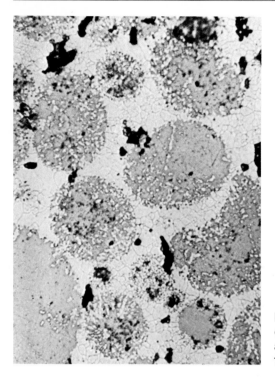

Fig. 15 Microstructures of a conventional composition dental amalgam. The $\gamma_2$ crystals are dispersed in the matrix. Probably no continuous network is formed.

The modified high copper amalgams deviate from the picture described for the conventional amalgams with respect to the $\gamma_2$ phase which either is absent or only present as a small percentage, provided the mercury content is not too high. Beyond a certain critical mercury content, which varies from alloy to alloy, most of the high copper amalgams, definitely contain the $\gamma_2$ phase (Jensen, 1977; Malhotra & Asgar, 1978). In case of the admixture type, tin liberated when mercury reacts with the $\gamma$ phase, reacts with copper from the silver-copper alloy particles to form $Cu_6Sn_5$. The $Cu_6Sn_5$ phase can be found in a reaction ring around the silver-copper particles (see fig. 17).

This reaction zone consists of both $Cu_6Sn_5$ and $\gamma_1$ phase (Okabe et al., 1977a; Mahler, Adey & Van Eysden, 1975; Vrijhoef & Driessens, 1973). A minor amount of $Cu_6Sn_5$ crystals is found in the matrix of the $\gamma_1$ phase (Okabe et al., 1977b) nucleated homogeneously from the mercury. Amalgams from high copper alloys of the all-in-one type show up no $\gamma_2$ phase either. Characteristic for this type amalgam likewise is the development of $Cu_6Sn_5$ crystals during hardening. In contrary with the admixture type, those crystals are found more frequently in the $\gamma_1$ matrix. Furthermore, $Cu_6Sn_5$ particles are formed on the surface of the amalgam alloy particles forming meshes. As pointed out by Okabe et al. (1977a; 1977b), probably, the $Cu_6Sn_5$ on the par-

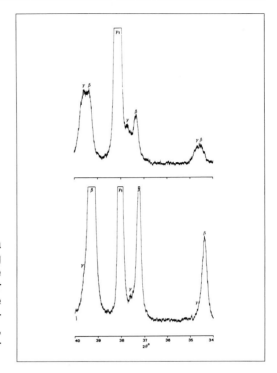

Fig. 16   X-ray diffraction patterns for a conventional composition amalgam showing the formation of the ternary Ag-Hg-Sn phase (the so-called $\beta_1$ phase). The upper and lower curve were measured after annealing the amalgam at 37°C for 1 day and 140 days respectively (according to Vrijhoef & Driessens, 1974, by permission of the Journal of Biomedical Materials Research).

ticle surface is formed before the $\gamma_1$ phase. They have proposed a dissolution-precipitation model giving at least a qualitative explanation as to the formation of reaction products. The results up to now suggest the reaction mechanisms of the amalgams from the admixture type of alloys to be different from those of the all-in-one type, because the $Cu_6Sn_5$ is formed in a continuous reaction layer around the silver–copper particles in case of the admixture type, whereas in case of the all-in-one alloys the $Cu_6Sn_5$ homogeneously precipitates from the liquid mercury.

From the work by *Aldinger & Kraft* (1977) it can be derived that for relatively high copper contents a copper-mercury phase can be expected as well. At this time, most of the questions as to the reaction mechanisms and resulting microstructure of the high copper amalgams still must be answered.

## 2.6. Porosity of the Amalgam

There are several factors contributing to the final porosity content of a set amalgam. We may distinguish between porosities due to manipulative variables and those originating in the nature of amalgam during setting.

Directly after trituration, empty spaces occur in the amalgam mix because of either insufficient trituration or too vigorous mixing. These porosities will be

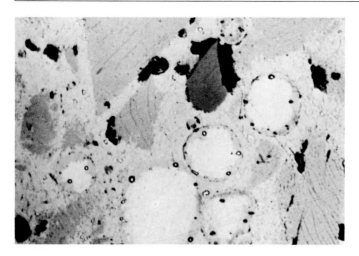

Fig. 17 Microstructure of a high copper amalgam of the admixture type.

eliminated completely or partially in the early stages of hardening directly after trituration under the influence of capillary forces by means of particle rearrangement and by the flow of liquid mercury into the porosities. Another manipulative factor substantially influencing the amount of porosity in a dental amalgam is the mode of condensation. It is obvious that careless condensation causes a lot of porosities, jeopardizing the properties of the amalgam.

Due to the hardening mechanism of dental amalgam, porosity is a more or less intrinsic feature of the material. The different processes giving rise to porosities might be summarized as follows. In case of hardening which is controlled by a dissolution-precipitation mechanism, there is a mass transport from the particles to the fluid, causing porosities in the original alloy particles. *Reynolds, Wawner & Wilsdorf* (1975) showed surface porosities to be filled by means of diffusion of $\gamma_1$ phase into these pores. So-called diffusion porosities, occurring at a greater dis-

tance from the alloy particle surface, probably will not be filled with $\gamma_1$ phase during the relatively short time during setting. After a certain time, the coalescing precipitates meet each other and sinter together. Porosities occur if this merging process is not completed.

As shown by *Aldinger* et al. (1976) mass transport of mercury into the alloy particles might cause porosities as well. Because of the diffusion of mercury into the solid alloy particles new phases are formed as a reaction ring around the particles making these particles swell. Although the particles might merge, this process can cause a substantial amount of porosity in amalgams with more silver than $Ag_3Sn$. The relative importance of the different processes for commercial amalgams is hardly known.

## 2.7. Structure of the Amalgam Surface

At the surface of a freshly set amalgam, original alloy particles can hardly be distinguished. This lack of representativity

30

of the surface layers for the amalgam as a whole can be explained from the fact that during trituration the amalgam alloy particles are wetted by mercury. Therefore, after hardening, these alloy particles are surrounded by reaction products with mercury. After polishing, a more representative amount of original alloy particles can be detected at the ground surface.

The outer surface of a freshly hardened amalgam is rough because crystals such as $\gamma_1$ and $\gamma_2$ phases grow at the surface (O'Brien, Johnston & Heinkel, 1977). Polishing gives a smoother surface and thus might be a valid recommendation for the clinical procedure.

## References

ADA (1968):
Guide to Dental Materials and Devices. 4th ed., American Dental Association, Chicago.

Aldinger, F., Schuler, P. & Petzow, G. (1976):
Reaktionsmechanismen beim Erhärten von Silber-Zinn-Amalgamen. Z. Metallk. **67,** 625.

Aldinger, F. & Kraft, W. (1977):
Über den Aufbau des Vierstoffsystems Silber-Kupfer-Zinn-Quecksilber bei 37°C. Z. Metallk. **68,** 523.

Asgar, K. (1974):
Amalgam Alloy with a Single Composition Behavior Similar to Dispersalloy. J. Dent. Res. **53,** Special Issue, paper 23.

Black, G. V. (1895):
An Investigation of the Physical Characters of the Human Teeth in Relation to their Diseases, and to Practical Dental Operations, Together with the Physical Characters of Filling-Materials. Third paper: Filling-Materials. Dent. Cosmos **37,** 553.

Black, G. V. (1896):
The Physical Properties of the Silver-Tin Amalgams. Dent. Cosmos **38,** 965.

Caul, H. J., Barton, J. A. & Manuszewski, R. C. 1968:
The Particle Size and Shape of Silver Alloys for Dental Amalgam. National Bureau of Standards Report No. 9984.

Innes, D. B. K. & Youdelis, W. V. (1963):
Dispersion Strengthened Amalgams. J. Can. Dent. Assoc. **29,** 587.

Jensen, S. J. (1972):
Copper-Tin Phase in Dental Silver Amalgam Alloy. Scand J. Dent. Res. **80,** 158.

Jensen, S. J., Andersen, P., Olesen, K. B. & Utoft, L. (1975):
The Location of Zinc in Dental Silver Amalgam. Scand. J. Dent. Res. **83,** 41.

Jensen, S. J. (1977):
Phase Content of a High Copper Silver Amalgam. Scand. J. Dent. Res. **85,** 297.

Johnson, L. B. (1971):
The Amount of Tin in the $\gamma_1$ Phase of Dental Amalgam. J. Biomed. Mater. Res. **5,** 239.

Johnson, L. B., Lawless, K. R., Stoner, G. E., Gardner, J., Young, R., Gerosky, T. R. Oppenheimer, E., Bender, S. T. & Neary, M. J. (1973):
Some Properties of Au-Containing Dental Amalgam. Biomater. Med. Devices Artif. Organs. **1,** 223.

Mahler, D. B., Adey, J. D. & Van Eysden, J. (1975):
Quantitative Microprobe Analysis of Amalgam. J. Dent. Res. **54,** 218.

Malhotra, M. L. & Asgar, K. (1978):
Investigation of Metallurgical Phases in High Copper Amalgams Containing Varying Mercury. J. Dent. Res. **57,** Special Issue A, paper 194.

Marshall, G. W., Finkelstein G. F. & Greener, E. H. (1975):
Microstructures of Several Cu Rich Dental Amalgams. J. Dent. Res. **54,** Special Issue A, paper 550.

Mitchell, R., Okabe, T. & Fairhurst, C. W. (1977):
The Effect of Dissolution of Silver-Tin Alloys on Amalgamation. J. Dent. Res. **56,** Special Issue B, paper 376.

Okabe, T., Hochmann, R. F. & Sims, L. O. (1975):
Amalgamation Reaction on Mercury-Plated Dental Alloy ($Ag_3Sn$). J. Biomed. Mater. Res. **9,** 221.

Okabe, T., Mitchell, R., Wright. A. H. & Fairhurst, C. W. (1977a):
Amalgamation on High Copper Single Composition Alloys. J. Dent. Res. **56,** Special Issue A, paper 146.

Okabe, T., Mitchel, R., Butts, M. B. & Fairhurst, C. W. (1977b):
Amalgamation Reaction of Dispersalloy and High Copper Single Composition Alloys. J. Dent. Res. **56,** Special Issue B, paper 378.

O'Brien, W. J., Johnston, W. M. & Heinkel, D. E. (1977):
Surface Properties of Dental Amalgam: Roughness Produced by Setting Reaction. J. Am. Dent. Assoc. **94,** 891.

Reynolds, C. L. & Barker, R. E. (1975):
Thermodynamic Consideration of the Setting Reaction in $Ag_3Sn$ Amalgams. J. Biomed. Mater. Res. **9,** 213.

Reynolds, C. L., Wawner, F. E. & Wilsdorf, H. G. F. (1975):
Amalgamation in the $Ag_3Sn$-Hg System. I. In Situ Observations. J. Appl. Physiol. **46,** 568.

Schoenmakers, H. P. L. (1967):
Toepassing van de F. D. I.-Specificatie op Enige in Nederland veel Gebruikte Amalgaamlegeringen. Ned. Tijdschr. Tandheelk. **74,** 1.

Shofu, Dental Corporation (1976):
Report on Indiloy.

Tobler, R. L., Rostoker, W. & Massler, M. (1974):
Development of a Ductile Dental Amalgam. J. Dent. Res. **53,** 907.

Vaidyanathan, T. K. & Greener, E. H. (1976):
Properties of a New Dental Amalgam Alloy Composition. J. Dent. Res. **55,** Special Issue B, paper 893.

Vrijhoef, M. M. A. (1973):
Dental Amalgam. An Explorative Study. Thesis, Nijmegen.

Vrijhoef, M. M. A. & Driessens, F. C. M. (1973):
X-Ray Diffraction Analysis of $Cu_6Sn_5$ Formation During Setting of Dental Amalgam. J. Dent. Res. **52,** 841.

Vrijhoef, M. M. A. & Driessens, F. C. M. (1974):
Long-Term Phase Changes in Dental Amalgam After Setting. J. Biomed. Mater. Res. **8,** 435.

Vrijhoef, M. M. A., Gubbels, G. H. M. & Driessens, F. C. M. (1975):
Creep of Dental Amalgam versus Composition and Prolonged Homogenization of Amalgam Alloy. Scripta Met. **9,** 85.

Vrijhoef, M. M. A. & Jensen, S. J. (1977):
Influence of the Heat Treatment of Commercial Amalgam Alloys on the Phase Composition of the Alloys and the Creep of the Resulting Amalgams. J. Biomed. Mater. Res. **11,** 339.

Waterstrat, R. M., Rupp, N. W. & Manuszweski, R. C. (1976):
Improved Creep Behavior and Removal of Gamma-2 Phase in Dental Amalgams Containing Manganese. J. Dent. Res. **55,** Special Issue B, paper 883.

# 3. Physical Properties of Dental Amalgam

## 3.1. Introduction

The ultimate lifetime of a dental amalgam restoration is determined by many factors having physical, chemical, biological, physiological and socio-economical aspects. In this chapter attention is only given to those aspects being directly related to the dental materials science.

In the first instance, four factors can be distinguished which play an important role in the initial lifetime expectancy of amalgam restorations: the material, the patient, the dentist as well as the service time under oral conditions.

Dominating factors in the early life of an amalgam restoration are the dentist and the material; the dentist, probably being the most important one. At this stage, the patient plays only a role of minor importance. As time proceeds, the restoration increasingly deteriorates under the aggressive oral influences up to the point that it must be replaced by a new restoration. An example of the influence of the factors amalgam alloy, patient and operator upon marginal fracture is depicted in fig. 18.

From this picture it is obvious that the influence of the amalgam alloy becomes more important, showing the "dynamic" character of the processes occurring under oral conditions. It must be stressed here that one should not generalize from fig. 18, because the re-presentativity of the different factors investigated is doubtful. For instance, the patients formed a rather uniform group as to the age, completeness of dentition, and other factors. Furthermore, only two dentists, who followed the same procedures, participated in the clinical trial. Therefore it might be expected that both the patient and operator effect will be of much more importance under general practice conditions.

Dental materials scientists express the quality aspects of amalgam restorations in terms of properties of the material. Initially, the properties of amalgam are determined by the composition and (micro) structure which, in their turn, are determined by the choice of the amalgam alloy and mercury, as well as their handling during the operative treatment. Unfortunately, this initial state is only transitory; the properties as well as the quality of the amalgam restoration deteriorates under the influence of the oral environment. As an example, the marginal deterioration of six different dental amalgams is shown in fig. 19.

The aim of this chapter is to describe the relevancy of certain properties for the functioning of amalgam restorations under oral conditions. Furhtermore, it will be dealt extensively with the importance of alloy choice and manipulation of the amalgam with respect to the quality of amalgam restorations. As far

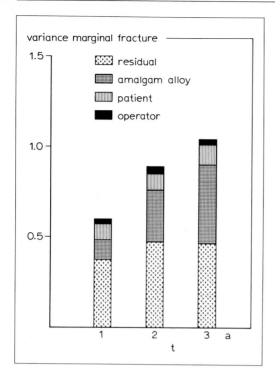

variance marginal fracture

- ▨ residual
- ▦ amalgam alloy
- ▥ patient
- ■ operator

Fig. 18    Analysis of components of the influence of the factors amalgam alloy, patient and operator upon marginal fracture as a function of the time under oral conditions (according to Letzel et al., 1978a).

as the manipulation is concerned, it will be attempted to specify its significance in case of both generally accepted clinical methods and modes of manipulation commonly referred to as bad practice. Aspects of amalgam manipulation will be further elaborated in chapter 5. Finally, repercussions of the properties of amalgam with respect to the cavity design will be quoted.

## 3.2. Dimensional Change

### 3.2.1. Relevancy of dimensional change

Dimensional change of a dental amalgam restoration is important with regard to its adaptation against the cavity wall.

A low degree of adaptation of a dental restoration to the cavity wall results in marginal leakage, which is assumed to be a condition for phenomena such as hypersensitivity, recurrent caries, pulpal damage, discoloration of the tooth as well as marginal breakdown of the amalgam restoration. It must be stressed here that the adaptation of an amalgam restoration against the cavity wall involves both adaptability and dimensional change. During condensation, the amalgam is pressed as well as possible against the cavity wall. At certain points, the restoration comes into contact with the cavity wall whereas at other positions an interspace between the restoration and the cavity wall occurs. The material on itself has a restricted ability to reproduce the

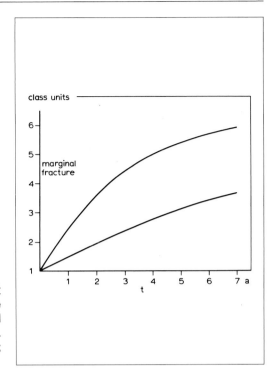

Fig. 19 Marginal fracture of two different dental amalgams as a function of the service time (in years) in the oral cavity (computed from Mahler, Terkla & Van Eysden, 1975). 20'th Century Micro Cut, upper curve; Dispersalloy, lower curve.

surface details of the cavity wall. Jørgensen (1965b) defined this ability as the adaptability of a direct restorative material. In case of an occlusal restoration, it is obvious that an expansion of the amalgam relative to the cavity results in more or less deformation of the initial geometric adaptation surface. A shrinkage will give a local loss of contact between the restoration and the cavity wall. However, the situation is much more complex, for instance, when the restoration is a MOD one. Then, a shrinkage might lead to a pressure against the axial walls, whereas local loss of contact might result at the lingual and buccal wall.

### 3.2.1.1. Dimensional change during hardening

In the early days of dental amalgam research, only expansion of amalgam was considered to be acceptable. More recently, both a slight expansion and contraction was considered to be acceptable because of both the uncertainty of the clinical importance as to the functioning and the undetectability by means of mirror and probe. However, systematic research data supporting these ideas are almost lacking. Combined clinical/laboratory research revealed that dimensional changes during hardening in the range from $-20$ µm/cm to $+20$ µm/cm are probably of no pertinence as to the marginal breakdown (see e. g. *Osborne*

*35*

et al., 1977; *Rupp, Pfaffenbarger & Manuszewski,* 1977; *Spanauf,* 1977). The existence of such a range around nil expansion c. q. contraction is quite reasonable, because other factors such as chewing forces and temperature changes also cause a fluctuating interspace between cavity wall and amalgam restoration. Forces exerted by the matrix band might play a role as well *(Bell,* 1977; *Powell, Nicholls & Shurtz,* 1977). Elastic deformations being produced when a Tofflemire matrix retainer is applied to a tooth range from 11.4 to 25.0 µm/cm *(Powell* et al., 1977). Removal of the matrix retainer gives a gap between cavity wall and restoration which is at least of the same order as a gap produced by a hardening contraction of 20 µm/cm. One might wonder whether dimensional change is clinically relevant. Probably, it is sufficient to mention that an extreme expansion during hardening might jeopardize occlusion and articulation, whereas the stresses, built up in the amalgam restoration and the tooth remnants, can lead to fracture of both tooth material and amalgam restoration. An exceptional contraction might give rise to caries around and underneath the restoration (see e. g. *Rupp* et al., 1977). Because most of the information as to the pertinence of dimensional change during hardening date from clinical investigations carried out more or less casuistically rather than systematically, the acceptable limits are not exactly known. However, it must be stressed here that the limits—20 µm/cm to + 20 µm/cm are probably safe limits. Unfortunately, leakage problems cannot be solved before a real adhesion between amalgam restoration and cavity wall is achieved by means of a coupling material.

### 3.2.1.2. Delayed expansion

As to the delayed expansion, probably major part of the dentists are aware of the problems involved. An example of a restoration showing up delayed expansion is given in fig. 20.

Condition for the occurrence of delayed expansion is the contamination with water (i. e. saliva, perspiration, etc.) of a zinc containing amalgam, which gives electrolytic corrosion. One of the products of this corrosion is hydrogen. Collection of hydrogen in the amalgam results in an internal pressure causing an excessive expansion (in the order of 500 µm/cm). For the patient the consequences are painful, and fracture of the tooth remnants or the amalgam restoration may occur. This reduces the functional lifetime of that particular restoration to a few weeks or months. In case of delayed expansion major problem for the dentist is that, at an early stage, it is almost undetectable on the basis of an extrusion of the restoration out of the cavity. This might be explained on the basis of both the rough surface of the cavity wall and the form of the cavity. *Jørgensen* (1977) has clearly demonstrated the influence of the surface condition of the cavity wall. Contaminated amalgam was condensed into artificial cavities made of glass. One cavity had a smooth surface, whereas the wall of the other one was rough. It was shown that an extreme expansion occurred in the cavity with the smooth surface. Almost no extrusion could be detected in case of the cavity with the rough surface. The latter artificial "tooth" broke into two pieces due to the great pressure exerted on the cavity wall. Indications as to the detection of delayed expansion at an early stage

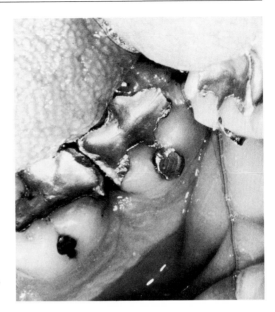

Fig. 20 A clinical case of delayed expansion.

may be tooth ache and blisters formed at the surface of the restorations.

### 3.2.2. Significance of materials choice and handling

*3.2.2.1. Dimensional change during hardening*

The setting expansions or contractions obtained from several commercially available dental amalgams are given in fig. 21.

Probably, the differences between the respective commercial dental amalgams are not clinically important as long as care is taken with regard to the proper handling of the materials according to currently accepted clinical rules (cf section 3.2.1.1.). At this time, it can be said that all specified alloys give reasonable results. Within the limits of the specification, no distinction can be made between the different amalgams.

However, it must be stressed here that the choice of an amalgam with a hardening expansion or contraction outside the present-day accepted levels might be dangerous (see e. g. *Rupp* et al., 1977). An illustration of the fact that generally accepted variations as to the handling of the materials probably have no clinically significant effect, is given in fig. 22.

However, there are (unacceptable) variations giving a very significant result. For instance, handling of the materials resulting in a high residual mercury content gives an unacceptable expansion (see fig. 23). In this case, the same clinical effects are involved as described for delayed expansion.

*3.2.2.2. Delayed expansion*

Whether the influence of the alloy is significant within the variations of accepted handling of the materials is

37

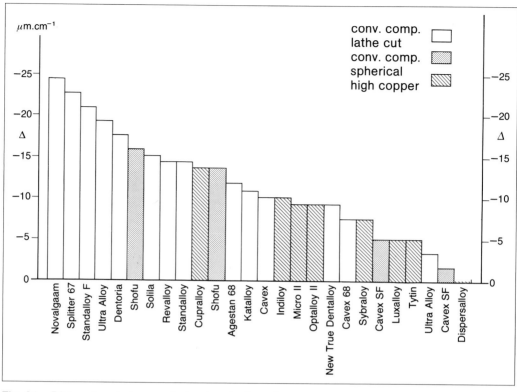

Fig. 21   Dimensional change during hardening of commercially available dental amalgams.

not clear. On a laboratory scale there are pronounced differences (cf section 4.3.). However, if contaminated with for instance saliva, all zinc containing amalgams show up unacceptable phenomena coupled with delayed expansion (what should be considered as "contamination" is dealt with in section 4.1.). It must be emphasized here that the contamination problems cannot be solved merely by the choice of a non-zinc alloy. Although the delayed expansion will not occur in such a case, the contamination will negatively affect the quality and stability of the amalgam through which the ultimate lifetime of the restoration will be reduced.

## 3.3. Strength

### 3.3.1. Pertinency of strength

For many dentists the strength problem is very clear. An amalgam restoration should be strong enough so as to resist the forces occurring in the oral cavity. Some even advocate: "the stronger, the better". Unfortunately, the situation is much more confusing because, especially during hardening, conflicting demands are made on the strength of dental amalgam.

### 3.3.1.1. Early-hour strength

Dental amalgam belongs to the so-called direct restorative materials. It is introduced into the prepared cavity as a

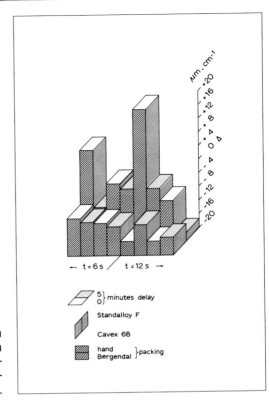

Fig. 22 Influence of the factors trituration time, amalgam alloy, delay time between mixing and condensing as well as condensation technic upon dimensional change during hardening (adapted from Spanauf, 1977).

plastic mass. However, this picture is only a transient one, for the setting reactions are active from the very beginning of trituration. After that time, the material develops its full strength in 8—24 hours (see fig. 24).

Frequently, the dental practitioner finds himself in need of time in order to finish completely the restoration before hardening. On the other hand sometimes, the dentist thinks that the amalgam never gets set. In the following part of this section attention will be paid to this confusing situation.

During condensation, the amalgam mass is expected to remain plastic. Strictly speaking, the dentist expects the material not to harden. Practically

speaking, the (ultimate) condensing time can be defined as the maximum time at which an amalgam without almost any pores can be obtained by means of a moderate condensation force.

At the time of the removal of the matrix band some resistance is assumed to be present, because the aim is not to jeopardize the form of the approximal parts of the restoration. Furthermore, no material should break away from these parts of the restoration during removal of the matrix band.

The amalgam should be sufficiently hardened to retain the form which is made during carving. At this stage, the material should not be pulled away from

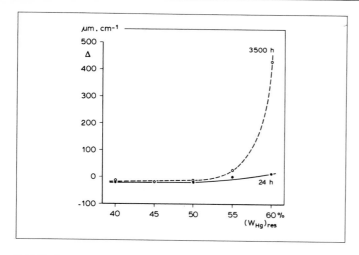

Fig. 23 Dimensional change $\Delta$ as a function of residual mercury content for annealing times of 24 and 3500 hours at 37°C (according to Vrijhoef, Spanauf & Driessens, 1975, by permission of the Australian Dental Journal.)

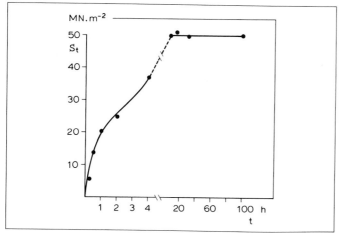

Fig. 24 Development of strength of a particular dental amalgam as a function of time.

the tooth structure because of a too high plasticity. However, because its carvability should be good, a refractory amalgam is undesirable at this stage. As shown by *Jørgensen & Isenoumi* (1969) the diametral tensile strength correlates significantly with the carvability: carvability decreases with increasing diametral tensile strength. It was the impression of *Jørgensen & Isenoumi* (1969) that the amalgam is no longer carvable when its diametral tensile strength is 3 MN/m² or more. The time to reach the point that the amalgam is not carvable any more might be referred to as the ultimate carving time. Other authors prefer a determination of the strength at a fixed time *(Ohashi, Ware & Docking,* 1975); *Kropp, Seyfried & Riethe,* 1977). Disadvantage of this method is that the dental practitioner has no clear insight into the actual time available for carving. During the occlusion determination, the restoration should be strong enough to minimize the risk of a fracture due to premature contact of the marginal ridges. However, some additional carving should be possible. In fig. 25 such a premature fracture is shown. This restoration was carved too high.

Apparently, the forces applied by the patient on the distal marginal ridge were fatal and the restoration was partially dislodged from the cavity. This problem is most important for quadrant dentistry (*Vermeersch,* 1975). Being dismissed from the dental chair, the patient is strongly advised to exert no masticatory forces for at least one or two hours after completion of the restoration. The rationality behind such an advise is obvious, at least qualitatively, from fig. 24. In order to have an indication of the risk of either a premature fracture or of a fracture shortly after dismissing the patient from the dental chair, it is obvious that at least the strength should be known between 15 and 60 minutes approximately. Irrespective of the influence of alloy choice and the handling of the materials, it should be stated that probably the most important factors as to the risk of a premature fracture are carving the restoration to an acceptable anatomical form and a controlled application of the force during the occlusion determination.

### 3.3.1.2. Strength after setting

The tensile strength after complete setting of the amalgam is recognized as a potential cause of failure of amalgam restorations subject to masticatory loading. This is particularly obvious in class II amalgam restorations. An example is shown in fig. 26.

In this case, tensile stresses at the isthmus area were responsible for the fracture of the restoration. Generally, such a gross fracture is a result of the compromise which has to be made. On the one hand the risk of the deterioration of the enamel and the dentin should be minimized; on the other hand a durable amalgam restoration should be obtained. Not always these conditions can be fulfilled simultaneously and as a result either the biologic material or the amalgam restoration will break. Satisfying these restraints was indeed a great problem in the period before and shortly after World War II (*Vrijhoef,* 1973).

However, as will be shown in the further part of this section, at this time there is no need for it any more. As far as a durable conservation of the biological remnants is concerned, it is obvious that the step cannot be prepared too wide or too deep. An extremely wide isthmus of a class II restoration might lead to fracture of the lingual or buccal walls, whereas a too deep step results in a possible pulp exposure. As far as the conditions are concerned to attain a durable amalgam restoration, it is just the other way round. The probability that isthmus fracture may occur, increases with decreasing depth and width of the step. This might be explained as follows. Several investigators have shown that during mastication tensile stresses occur at the isthmus area (see e. g. *Mahler,* 1958). The reaction stresses due to mastication have to be distributed over the cross section at the isthmus. Because stress equals force over area, therefore, the smaller this cross section the higher the stress. Thus, as a result, an increase of either the width or the depth of the step gives a lower probability of the occurrence of isthmus fracture. The generally accepted cavity design of a class II preparation obviously is a balance between a reasonable durability of both the rem-

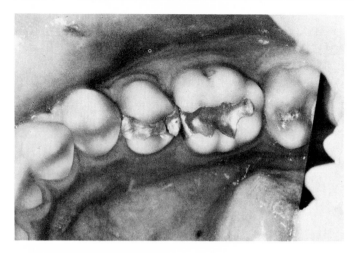

Fig. 25 Fractured amalgam restoration due to premature contact during the determination of occlusion and articulation.

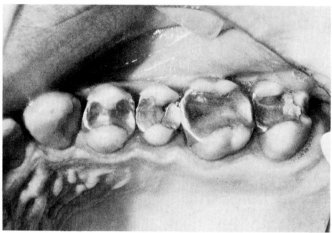

Fig. 26 Clinical case of a gross fracture due to insufficient bulk at the isthmus (according to Vrijhoef, Vermeersch & Spanauf, 1979, by permission of the Editor of the Journal of Oral Rehabilitation).

nants of the tooth structures and the amalgam restoration. Dissection of the restoration depicted in fig. 26 showed the step to be inadequate in depth. For that patient a more adequate cavity was prepared. It has been functioning now statisfactorily in the oral cavity for some years (as for the demonstration of the importance of cavity design for the occurrence of gross fracture see e. g. *Nadal, Phillips & Swartz*, 1961b). The tensile strength of hardened amalgam is a pertinent property with regard to some other aspects related to the activities of the general practitioner as well. For instance, modelling an amalgam restoration, only a very superficial pit and fissure pattern is made rather than a detailed one. This might be explained on a basis of the fact that investigations have shown the tensile stress to be a maximum at the surface of the class II restoration. A very detailed pit and fissure carving gives higher tensile stresses as well as stress concentrations. This might start the fracture of the restoration. Apart from mechanically inclined considerations, other factors play a role as to the decision not to make a very detailed pit and fissure carving either. Both pits and fissures are ideal accumalation positions for food debris. Corrosion will mainly start in these areas and thereby attack the restoration and jeopardize the functional aspects of the amalgam restoration. Corrosion leads to another problem. Up to now, attention has been only paid to the probability of the occurrence of isthmus fracture of a rather freshly set amalgam. However, as time proceeds strength decreases because the amalgam restoration deteriorates under the influence of the oral environment. It is clear that for amalgams (heavily) corroded under service conditions, the strength in corroded condition plays a more dominant role than the "fresh" strength.

### 3.3.2. Importance of materials choice and handling

#### 3.3.2.1. Early-hour strength

If the dental practitioner sticks to the manipulative limits given by the different manufacturers it is reasonable that the factor amalgam alloy is the most important one with regard to the clinical functioning. This might be judged from fig. 27 based upon the work by Spanauf, Vermeersch & Vrijhoef (1976a). In this study, the influence of the factors amalgam alloy (8 alloys), trituration technique (hand mixing versus trituration by means of an amalgamator) and the mode of packing (hand packing versus condensation with a mechanical vibrator) upon the tensile strength was investigated.

From fig. 27 it is clear that the differences between the amalgams are much more pronounced than those between the trituration and condensation techniques respectively. Probably, good results (i. e. sufficient enough) as to the early-hour strength can be obtained with a variety of technics, as long as no bad practice is carried out. Because the amalgam alloy probably is so important, it is interesting to explore further the influence of this factor. Furthermore, some attention will be given to the influence of the hardening time. Fig. 28 provides this information. From this figure the differences between the distinct amalgams are apparent. The influence of the hardening time is obvious as well. There is a tendency that an amalgam giving a relatively high tensile strength after 15 minutes also gives a relatively high strength after 30 or 60 minutes.

At this moment, only provisional conclusions can be drawn as to the factor alloy. True, amalgams with the highest strength values can be selected. For example, after 15 minutes Indiloy, one of the Cavex SF alloys, Micro II, Optalloy II and Revalloy reveal to have amalgams showing up the highest diametral tensile strength values. After 60 minutes amalgams from Indiloy, the two Cavex SF alloys, Micro II, Optalloy II as well as the two Shofu alloys turn out to be the best. Self-evident, the 2 MN/m$^2$ requirement after 15 minutes of the former ADA specification no. 1 might be used as well: 13 of the 23 amalgams satisfy this requirement. However, the conflicting demands should be satisfied too. If we take, for instance, a diametral tensile strength of 3 MN/m$^2$ as a critical level for an acceptable carving, several amalgams should be amply

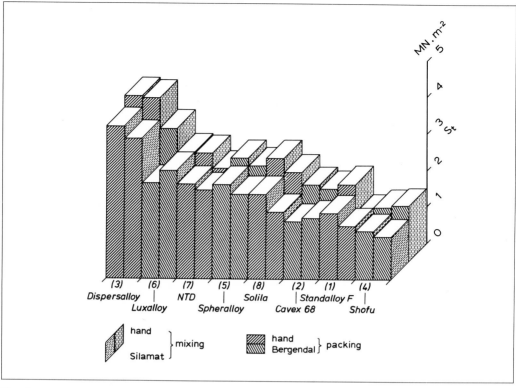

Fig. 27   Influence of the factors amalgam alloy, trituration technique and mode of packing upon the 15-minutes tensile strength (data from Spanauf, Vermeersch & Vrijhoef, 1976a).

carved within 15 minutes. Last years, there has been a demand from general practitioners for (very) quick setting amalgams. Consequently, some of the modern amalgams are setting at a very high rate with the result that some dentists and most of the dental students cannot cope with this situation.

### 3.3.2.2. Strength after setting

As to the question whether the factors amalgam alloy and manipulation of the amalgam significantly influence the tensile strength, and thereby the functioning of amalgam restorations under oral conditions, the following statement will

be clarified: "Almost no isthmus fractures will be observed if generally accepted rules with respect to cavity preparation and amalgam manipulation are taken into consideration. Less than 1% approximately of the amalgam restorations will show up isthmus fracture within a two years period".

This statement is explained by means of fig. 29 as far as the factor alloy choice is concerned, which is constructed on the basis of the work by *Vrijhoef, Vermeersch & Spanauf* (1979); diametral tensile strength values of 23 amalgams are given. The differences between the amalgams are obvious. The range of

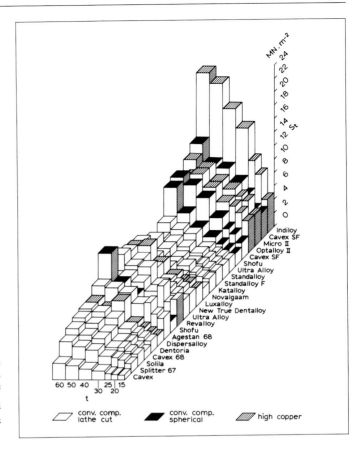

Fig. 28 Influence of the amalgam alloy and the setting time upon the strength of the hardening amalgam (data from Spanauf, Vermeersch & Vrijhoef, 1976b).

diametral tensile strength values is from 37—56 MN/m$^2$ approximately. At the 55th general session of the IADR in Copenhagen, *Asgar, Arfaei & Mahler* (1977) showed that the diametral tensile test might be an underestimation of the true tensile strength, especially for amalgam showing up a relatively low creep.

If we take this effect into consideration the high risk amalgams are those having a relatively high creep and/or low diametral tensile strength.

The high creep amalgams are Novalgaam, Splitter 67, Standalloy F and Luxalloy. Relatively low diametral ten-sile strength values are obtained for Revalloy, Cavex 68, Cavex, Dispersalloy, Luxalloy, Solila, Optalloy II and Micro II. The highest risk has Luxalloy which might have a tensile strength that is of the order of 35 MN/m$^2$. It might be asked whether the amalgams having a relatively bad expectation in the laboratory give real high risk restorations as to the bulk fracture occurring under oral conditions. The answer is definitely "no" as long as care is taken of an adequate cavity design and proper materials handling. This answer can be based on the following facts. Several of the amalgams with a relatively bad la-

45

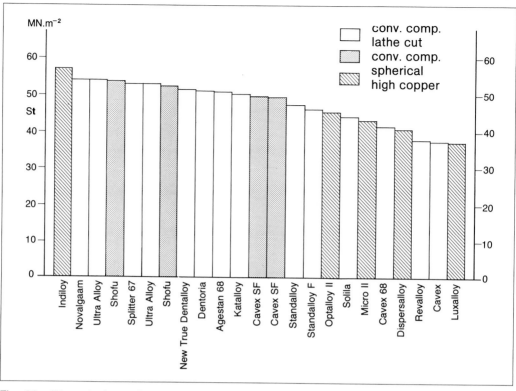

Fig. 29  Diametral tensile strength of 23 commercial dental amalgams (computed from Vrijhoef, Vermeersch & Spanauf, 1979).

boratory expectation are used in a clinical study. For instance, in simultaneous research projects at the University of Nijmegen and the University of Louvain, among others, high risk amalgams from Standalloy F, Luxalloy, Dispersalloy and Optalloy II are under investigation. In these projects, amalgams with a low risk are incorporated as well. Almost no gross fractures are reported (see e. g. *Letzel* et al., 1977). Neither for the group of amalgams with a good prospect nor for those having a bad expectation. In other clinical trials bulk fracture is not reported at all or only a few tenths of a percent of the total number of restorations.

Practically speaking, one might conclude that if the choice is made for an alloy as required by a dental specification it is highly unlikely that the restoration will fail as far as the alloy is concerned. The question still remains whether the influence of the manipulation of the amalgam is clinically important. The statement which will be elucidated is: "If the dentist keeps within the limits prescribed by the manufacturers and described in dental text books almost no isthmus fracture or other detrimental effect related to tensile strenght can be observed." It is sufficient to put forward that in the clinical research projects in Nijmegen, Woluwé and many other places, different clinicians with a different background and divergent manipulative abilities have placed the dental amalgam restorations. In some projects also students have cooperated. In all those projects hardly any isthmus fracture or other negative phenomena related to tensile strength could be found. On this basis, therefore, it is safe to conclude that the probability of the occurrence of isthmus fracture is practically speaking nil if the dental team adheres to a generally accepted manipulation of the material. In case if a too high percentage of isthmus fractures, for instance 5%, is observed the dentist should try to answer the following questions:

— Does the amalgam satisfy a dental specification?
— Is the cavity preparation done according to the appropriate rules?
— Is the amalgam manipulation carried out adequately?

On the basis of this section it might be strongly advised not to overestimate the importance of strength after setting as advertized by manufacturers: one amalgam being even stronger than another one. Probably all, at least the certified products, are strong enough as long as the factor dentist (cavity preparation, materials handling) is properly controlled. At this time the range of tensile strength values of the available commercial amalgams probably is not large enough to permit the dentist to prepare the cavity beyond the accepted limits of present day cavity design.

## 3.4. Creep

### 3.4.1. Relevancy of creep

In designing machines or constructions to be operated at high temperatures, engineers need to have a thorough knowledge as to the creep resistance of materials at these temperatures. Designers in the chemical and power generating industry are quite familiar with the concept of an estimate of the functional lifetime of a part of a construction on the basis of its creep behaviour.

The basis of their technique can be explained by means of the creep curve given in fig. 30.

After the creep load is applied at zero time, an instantaneous elastic deformation occurs. Then there is the so-called transient creep or stage 1 creep. During stage 2 creep, or steady-state creep, the dependence of deformation on time can be represented by a straight line. During stage 3 the process accelerates till the amalgam breaks down. This will happen in a relatively short time. If the times of stage 1 and stage 3 were neglected, the time till fracture would be determined by stage 2. As a first approximation this is a reasonable assumption (see e. g. *Jongenburger*, 1977). The time of stage 2 is inversely proportional to the steady-state creep (the steady-state creep is the slope of the creep curve at stage 2). As mentioned before, creep problems occur at relatively high temperatures. Although service temperatures under oral conditions are not high, it can be expected that dentists are confronted with the creep problem in case of amalgam restorations. From technical literature it is known that the creep of a material

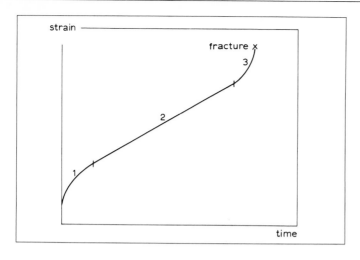

Fig. 30 A schematic creep curve (by permission of the Australian Dental Journal).

plays an important role at a service temperature ($T_s$) higher than about half the melting temperature ($T_m$). As in the case of dental amalgam $T_s/T_m \sim 310/350\,K \sim 0.9$, the expectation of a creep problem at mouth temperature is justified by theory. Recently, indications of such a problem were found in the field of dental amalgam restorations. *Mahler* et al. (1970) reported a correlation between creep and the susceptibility of dental amalgam restorations to marginal fracture: a higher creep corresponds with more marginal breakdown. As known from clinical studies, marginal breakdown of amalgam restorations is one of the most frequently occurring failures under oral conditions (see fig. 31). The correlation between creep and marginal fracture was confirmed by several other investigators (see e. g. *Mahler, Van Eysden & Terkla*, 1975; *Vrijhoef*, 1975; *Letzel* et al., 1977; *Osborne* et al., 1977b; *Osborne* et al., 1978).

This correlation attracts a lot of attention in advertizing and in publications. Frequently, statements can be found expressing either explicitly or implicitly that a low creep amalgam would solve the marginal fracture problem. In the following part of this section an attempt will be made to show that such a statement is not necessarily correct.

In fig. 32 marginal fracture is plotted against creep. These observations were taken from two publications by *Osborne* et al. (1977b, 1978). Unfortunately, technical problems (e. g. another creep test) prevented to include data obtained by other investigators.

Marginal fracture is expressed in terms of the so-called ridits. It is not wihtin the scope of this section to explain these ridits. However, the higher the ridits the more marginal breakdown. In fig. 32 it has been distinguished between two groups of amalgams. The dots represent the $\gamma_2$ free amalgams, whereas the open circles correspond with conventional composition, and therefore with $\gamma_2$ containing amalgams. Two amalgams are suggested to be $\gamma_2$ free. However, effectively these two amalgams belong to the group of $\gamma_2$ containing amalgams.

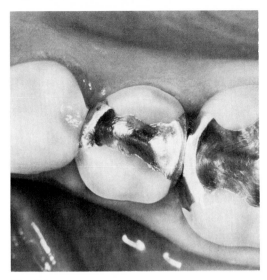

Fig. 31 a

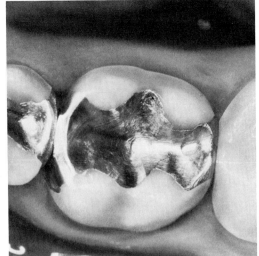

Fig. 31 b

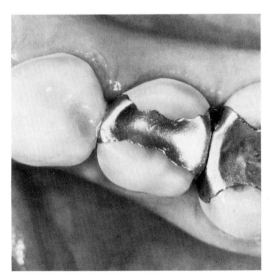

Fig. 31 c

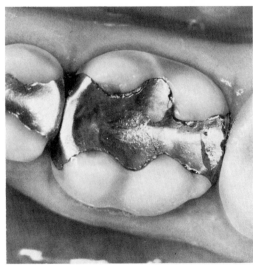

Fig. 31 d

Fig. 31 Two amalgam restorations in the same oral cavity after polishing (a and b) and two years later (c and d). The difference between the marginal fracture of the two restorations illustrates the influence of the factor alloy (Courtesy of Dr. H. Letzel).

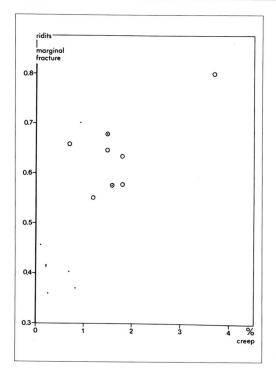

Fig. 32 Marginal fracture as a function of creep for several dental amalgams (computed from Osborne et al., 1977b and 1978).

These amalgams are given as circles with a dot inside. If one takes the group as a whole it is clear that there is a correlation between marginal fracture and creep. However, there are several exceptions proving the rule. Therefore, it is questionable whether this correlation is a good basis for using creep as a selection criterion to buy an alloy. An analysis of fig. 32 reveals that a wrong decision would be taken in 33% of all possibilities. Thus in 33% of the possible decisions based on the creep the worst amalgam instead of the best would be selected. Although the negative consequences of such a wrong decision are not always serious as far as the marginal fracture is concerned, one might doubt whether the creep is as important as some manufacturers suggest. At any rate, this is clear in case if one selects an alloy from the group of $\gamma_2$ free amalgams. Inspection of fig. 32 already reveals that there is no significant correlation between marginal breakdown and creep. This bad correlation corresponds with a large number of wrong decisions; more than 60% would be faulty. In case of the $\gamma_2$ containing amalgams the situation is slightly better. For this group one gets 50% of wrong decisions approximately.

Analysis of the literature data reveals the correlation of marginal fracture with creep probably to hold true for the group of $\gamma_2$ containing amalgams. From the available clinical investigations only those by *Mahler* et al. (1975), *Letzel* et al. (1977), *Osborne* et al. (1977b) and *Rupp* et al. (1977) report about a sufficient number of conventional composition amalgams (5, 5, 6 and 6 $\gamma_2$ containing amalgams respectively). Statistical testing of the data reported by *Mahler* et al. (1975) and *Rupp* et al. (1977) by means of a test of Spearman reveals a positive correlation between creep and marginal fracture. Analysis of the data by *Letzel* et al. (1977b) gives an indication for a positive correlation whereas no correlation could be found for the data reported by *Osborne* et al. (1977b). Apart from the publications by *Osborne* et al. (1977b, 1978), no other suitable literature data are present for the group of $\gamma_2$ free amalgams. However, on the basis of their results it should be concluded that no correlation between creep and marginal deterioration is present for the $\gamma_2$ free amalgams. It might be astonishing why the creep-marginal fracture correlation holds true justifiably in the case that no distinction between $\gamma_2$ containing and $\gamma_2$ free amalgams is made. It is not within the scope of the present section to solve this problem. However, it might be caused by the fact that two different groups of amalgams were chosen. More research is necessary to clarify this and other questions. Investigators have made attempts to describe marginal deterioration at a theoretical level as well. The most attention is given to a theory by *Jørgensen* (1965a), which is referred to as the so-called mercuroscopic theory. Because corrosion is the main element of his theory it will be dealt with in section 3.5.1. Up to now, the correlation between creep and marginal deterioration is not at all or hardly explained in terms of a cause and effect relationship. *Dérand* (1977) indicated how creep might play a role in the model of *Jørgensen*. On the basis of computa-

tions of the stresses induced in a class II restoration loaded at the cusps, *Dérand* (1977) showed that the resulting creep might cause a narrow defect between the amalgam and the tooth, which might lead to a film of saliva in the interspace and therefore to an accelerated corrosion, which is the main cause of marginal fracture in the mercuroscopic theory. *Vrijhoef* (1975) pointed out that for the group of conventional amalgams interaction of creep with corrosion might play a role as well. It was made clear that amalgams prone to corrosion probably reveal a high creep. From the theories published up to now it is not clear what role creep is playing in the processes behind the marginal fracture.

As far as the creep—marginal fracture correlation is concerned it might be concluded that there is probably a correlation between creep and marginal breakdown for the conventional $\gamma_2$ containing amalgams. However, there is probably no correlation for the $\gamma_2$ free amalgams. It might be useful to conclude not to overestimate creep as a selection criterion for the alloy to predict marginal fracture, because more than 60% wrong decisions might be taken. Clinical evidence is more reliable. Finally, it must be concluded that the role of creep in the marginal breakdown mechanism is not clear.

### 3.4.2. Significance of materials choice and handling

The influence of the factor amalgam alloy upon creep is very important. The creep values of several commercial amalgams are given in fig. 33.
As shown in section 3.4.1. for the group

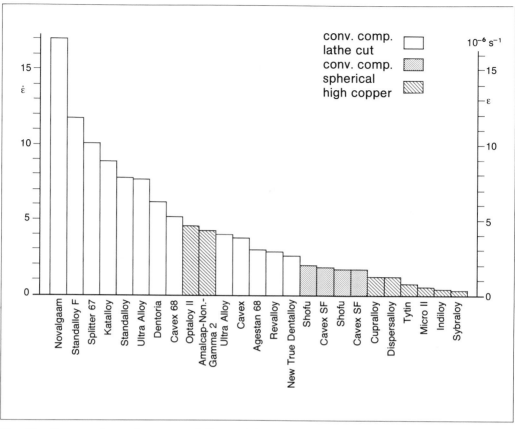

Fig. 33   Creep values of commercially available dental amalgams.

of "conventional composition" amalgams, the creep can be used as a first approximate predictor of marginal breakdown under oral conditions. Because no acceptable levels are known for marginal fracture, specification of the maximum allowable creep level is more or less arbitrary. It is strongly advised not to use creep as an indicator for marginal fracture for the $\gamma_2$-free amalgams. From fig. 33 it is obvious that the influence of the factor alloy upon creep is evident for this group of amalgams. However, other factors unknown at this moment should be taken into account to construct a reasonable predictor for marginal fracture.

From laboratory studies it is known that the handling of materials can have a substantial influence upon the creep. Some examples are given in fig. 34 and fig. 35.

These figures are self-explanatory as far as the influence upon creep is concerned. However, they do not produce any evidence as to their clinical interpretation. At this time, hardly any information is available from combined clinical/laboratory research. *Osborne* et al. (1977a) have reported about the in

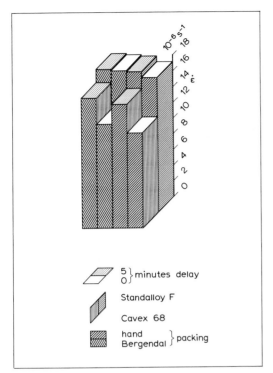

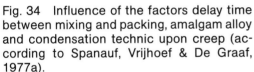

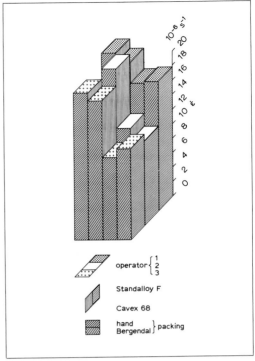

Fig. 34   Influence of the factors delay time between mixing and packing, amalgam alloy and condensation technic upon creep (according to Spanauf, Vrijhoef & De Graaf, 1977a).

Fig. 35   Influence of the factors operator, amalgam alloy and packing technic upon creep (according to Spanauf, Vrijhoef & De Graaf, 1977b).

fluence of the factor trituration time upon creep. A schematic presentation of a typical curve from their study is given in fig. 36.

At first, the results reported by *Osborne et al.* (1977a) show up a decrease of creep with increasing mixing time. By further increasing the trituration time, they have shown the creep to increase too. Thereby, they illustrated that an optimum mixing time might exist. *Osborne & Gale* (1974b) have found indications that creep differences due to different trituration times are correlated with marginal fracture, similarly as found by other investigators for creep variations caused by the choice of another amalgam alloy. However, they did their experiments with only one amalgam. More research is necessary to clarify whether this correlation holds true for other amalgams. Although at this moment the clinical significance of the influence of manipulative variables upon creep is unknown the results can be used at least qualitatively. For it is known that more creep of a particular amalgam corresponds with an inferior microstructure. Although the extent of the clinical

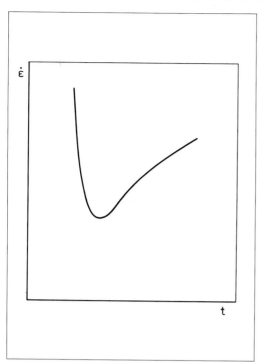

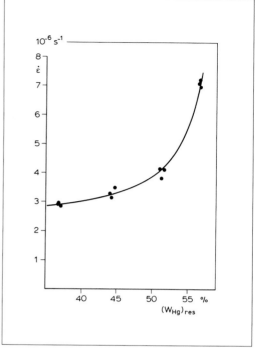

Fig. 36 Schematic representation of the influence of trituration time upon creep (analogously to Osborne et al., 1977 a).

Fig. 37 The influence of the residual mercury content upon the creep of a particular amalgam.

significance of these changes is unknown, it is wise to avoid such a situation. For example, it is known that the influence of mercury content upon creep has the form as given in fig. 37.

For a low mercury content creep is rather independent of mercury content. However, if the mercury content exceeds 55—60 wt.% dramatic changes occur. Not only creep but other properties such as dimensional change and strength show up undesirable changes also in that range of mercury contents. Dentists should take care to avoid such a region because it is known to be a misuse of the material. More scientific work is necessary in order to find out whether even the slightest changes occurring within the accepted range of mercury contents have significant consequences for oral conditions.

## 3.5. Tarnish and Corrosion

### 3.5.1. Pertinence of tarnish and corrosion

A well known and frequently recognized phenomenon in the early life of an amalgam restoration is the "galvanic pain" due to the galvanic action of amalgam restorations in combination with other metallic restorations (see e. g. *Nachlin*, 1954; *Fusayama, Katayori & Nomoto*,

1963; *Marxkors, 1970*). In a casuistic clinical study *Mumford* (1960) found that this type of pain occurred only in a small percentage of cases. Further, he found the pain to be not so serious generally. It occurred usually in the first hours and in no instance did it last longer than for a few weeks after the insertion of the material. It has also been mentioned by several authors that the galvanic current could have a harmful effect on the soft oral tissues or on the human organism as a whole. However, the frequency of the occurrence of these effects is supposed to be low or absent as reported by several authors (see e. g. *Phillips*, 1957; *Fusayama* et al., 1963).

The loss of luster and aesthetic quality, which has been reported by several authors *(Phillips* et al., 1945; *Nadal* et al., 1961a & b; *Wilson & Ryge,* 1963; *Mathewson, Brunner & Noonan,* 1967; *Duperon, Nevile & Kasloff,* 1977; *Watson* et al., 1973; *Letzel* et al., 1978 a en b), are the first indications as to the deteriorating surface of the amalgam restoration and the bulk of the material underneath. Although tarnish (see fig. 38) is no failure in itself, generally it heralds a more severe form of corrosion (see fig. 39). A rough surface of the amalgam restoration is prone to the formation of plaque and causes the irritation to the adjacent soft tissues if in contact with the latter. Penetration of corrosion in the bulk of the amalgam restoration weakens its structure which results in a substantial loss of strength. As already remarked by *Schoonover & Souder* (1941) this corrosion can be so severe that the amalgam obtained from some extracted teeth "had apparently lost much of its strength and could be crumbled between the fingers".

*Schoonover & Souder* (1941) pointed out that the corrosion products cause a discoloration of the dentine which can be clinically observed (see also *Hals* et al, 1975).

The corrosion products coming out of the restoration also might have a positive effect. If precipitated in the interspace between cavity wall and restoration, less saliva can penetrate into it. As a result, the restoration can be sealed *(Phillips* et al., 1961). Moreover, it should be stressed that local corrosion is the main cause of delayed expansion (see section 3.2.).

Up to now, it was dealt with corrosion under oral conditions. It would be not out of place to pay attention to laboratory experiments with regard to corrosion. Unfortunately, at this time no reliable corrosion test is available. One of the factors influencing the absence of such a good test might be the fact that one single test can never predict the variety of aspects of corrosion occurring in the oral cavity. Therefore, care should be taken as to the interpretation of corrosion tests carried out under laboratory conditions.

As already mentioned in section 3.4.1. *Jørgensen* (1965a) assumes corrosion to be the driving force for the mechanism undermining the marginal areas of restorations made from conventional composition amalgams. *Jørgensen* (1965a) made a distinction between fracture caused by pressure (p-type) and fracture caused by pull (t-type). It is clear that both types of forces are exerted on the free surface of the restoration (for instance pressure exerted by chewing and pull due to adhesion of a caramel). By examining amalgam restorations in extracted teeth he found that the p-type fracture occurred most

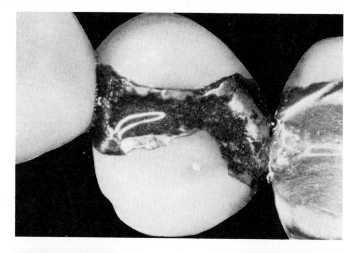

Fig. 38   A clinical example of a tarnished amalgam restoration.

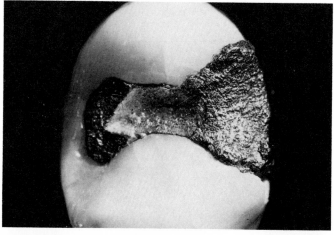

Fig. 39 a

Fig. 39 b

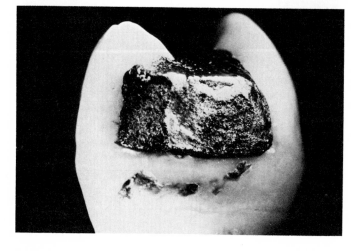

Fig. 39   A clinical example of a corroded amalgam restoration.

(a) An occlusal view.

(b) The approximal part of the restoration.

frequently. In the following discussion, therefore, we will restrict ourselves to the p-type of marginal breakdown.

Jørgensen postulated corrosion of the $\gamma_2$ phase to be the cause. The circumstances between cavity wall and restoration promote corrosion of the $\gamma_2$ phase, which is accompanied by a release of mercury. This mercury reacts with the remnants of the particles of the amalgam alloy. This process is followed by the so-called mercuroscopic expansion of the amalgam adjacent to the cavity wall, resulting in an unsupported wedge at the margin of the restoration. Because of the relative weakness of this wedge, originating in the microstructure of the amalgam (high mercury content and the presence of a lot of porosities due to corrosion) as well as the structural weakness of the wedge (weaker for the smaller cavo-surface angles), marginal breakdown is possible under the influence of the forces in the oral cavity. The theory of *Jørgensen* is one of the arguments to prepare a cavo-surface angle of 90° as well as possible. *Dérand* (1977) indicated how creep might play a role in the model of Jørgensen. On the basis of computations of the stresses induced in a class II restoration loaded at the cusps, *Dérand* (1977) showed that the resulting creep might cause a narrow defect between the amalgam and the tooth. This space not adapted to the margin might lead to a film of saliva in the interspace and therefore to an accelerated corrosion. Theoretically, besides the interspace formation as pointed out by *Dérand* (1977), an increase of the size of the cavity relative to the restoration, originating for example in temperature changes, chewing forces or hardening contraction might give access to saliva at the interspace between dentinal wall and amalgam restoration. *Vrijhoef* (1975) pointed out that interaction of creep with corrosion might play a role as well. It was made clear that amalgams prone to corrosion probably reveal a high creep because they depend upon the same microstructural features. *Granath & Hiltscher* (1970) investigated the stress distribution in class II restorations, assuming a perfect marginal adaptation of the restoration to the tooth. They found that loading of the edge can cause fracture without the load per unit area having exceeded the maximum compressive strength of the amalgam. It is obvious that their conclusions should be taken in addition to those of *Jørgensen* (1965a) especially in case of either a heavily corroded amalgam margin or the one with a relatively high mercury content.

From the theories described above, no clear picture of the reality can be derived because much of the experimental evidence is lacking. A lot of verification work still should be done in this respect.

### 3.5.2. Significance of materials choice and handling

One aspect of the theory according to *Jørgensen* (1965a) gets a lot of attention in both advertisements and publications in the journals; especially after the introduction of the $\gamma_2$ free amalgams. Often a statement can be found suggesting that an elimination of the $\gamma_2$ phase from dental amalgam solves the marginal breakdown problem. In the following part of this section an attempt will be made to show that this statement is not correct and may be misleading. Several clinical investigators have reported marginal breakdown data for two or more commercial amalgams (Wilson & Ryge, 1963; Mahler et al., 1970; Weaver et al., 1970; Duperon et al., 1971; Mahler, Terkla & Van Eysden, 1973; Binon et al., 1973; Mathewson, Retzlaff & Porter, 1974; Osborne & Gale, 1974a; Mahler et al., 1975; Osborne et al., 1976; Charbeneau, Bozell & Carpenter, 1977; Leinfelder et al., 1977b; Rupp et al., 1977; Sockwell, Leinfelder & Taylor, 1977; Letzel et al., 1978 a and b; Osborne et al., 1978). The susceptibility to marginal deterioration of the respective commercial amalgams has been deduced from these data and is displayed in fig. 40. It must be stressed here that a strict quantitative interpretation of these data is not allowed because of methodological differences between the investigations, batch differences, differences of handling materials, differences between patients, and other factors. At the present moment it is clear for instance that (20th Century) Micro Cut gives much more marginal fracture than Dispersalloy. However, problems arise when the heights of the columns equal each other approximately. For instance, one should be careful if (20th Century) Fine Cut is compared with New True Dentalloy. In this case differences between dentists, patients and other factors play a role as well. One should be careful as far as the quantitative interpretation of fig. 40 is concerned.

Spheraloy and Tytin are displayed at several places in this figure because contradictory data were found in literature. In case of Spheraloy, these differences probably are caused by batch differences. A relatively bad reproducibility of some clinical experiments might play a role as well. The smaller differences as reported in the case of Tytin might originate in batch differences of both Tytin and Dispersalloy with which it was compared in two different studies. The different Dispersalloy batches used in clinical investigations up to now, were produced by four different manufacturers. Laboratory studies of batches of the present-day product manufactured by Johnson & Johnson indicate batch differences to play a role for this amalgam as well (see e. g. Darvell, 1976).

In fig. 40 a distinction is made between lathe cut alloys of conventional composition, spherical alloys of conventional composition as well as high copper alloys. Most of the high copper amalgams might be considered to be $\gamma_2$ free. However, amalgams from Micro II and Optaloy II contain a considerable amount of $\gamma_2$ phase. At best, these amalgams can be referred to as $\gamma_2$ reduced. Fig. 40 clearly illustrates that some of the non-$\gamma_2$ amalgams belong to the best amalgams as far as marginal fracture is concerned. Some others such as Sybraloy and Aristaloy CR show up a relatively large amount of marginal fracture. Micro II and Optaloy II which might be considered to be $\gamma_2$ reduced amalgams, apparently do not show up a superior marginal integrity either. Therefore, it may be provisionally, concluded that marginal fracture problems are not automatically solved by either a $\gamma_2$ free or a $\gamma_2$ reduced amalgam. In order to make it possible to solve the marginal fracture at a theoretical level it might be necessary to take into account more than one type of marginal fracture (cf Jørgensen, 1965a). Furthermore, it is advisable to take into account more than one property rather than only creep or corrosion.

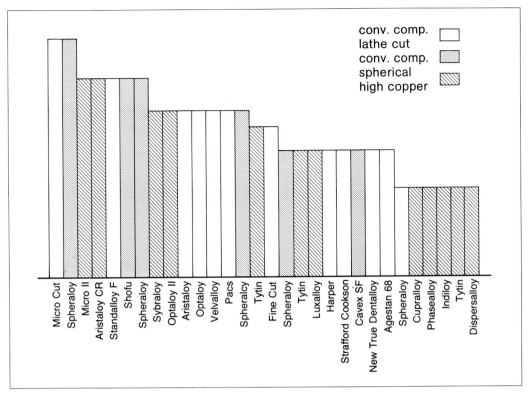

conv. comp.
lathe cut
conv. comp.
spherical
high copper

Micro Cut
Spheraloy
Micro II
Aristaloy CR
Standalloy F
Shofu
Spheraloy
Sybraloy
Optaloy II
Aristaloy
Optaloy
Velvalloy
Pacs
Spheralcy
Tytin
Fine Cut
Spheraloy
Tytin
Luxalloy
Harper
Strafford Cookson
Cavex SF
New True Dentalloy
Agestan 68
Spheraloy
Cupralloy
Phasealloy
Indiloy
Tytin
Dispersalloy

Fig. 40    The susceptibility to marginal breakdown of some commercial amalgams (derived from several clinical trials; for references see text).

The question remains for the general practitioner: which alloy to choose as far as marginal deterioration is concerned? The answer is not a simple one. First of all, it might be put forward that fig. 40 is based upon rather short-term investigations. Up to date, the admissible amount of marginal fracture in the long run is completely unknown. In the preceding section it has been already stated that comparing the amalgams quantitatively is difficult because of batch differences, patient effects, and other factors. Therefore, selecting a critical marginal fracture level is more or less arbitrary in practice. The authors of the present work would like to take the limit at a height of the group of New True Dentalloy. The reason for this selection lies in the fact that this alloy has been in use for long time with a relatively good experience in many dental schools. Therefore, as far as marginal fracture is concerned one might select for instance New True Dentalloy, Cavex SF, Luxalloy or Dispersalloy or an equivalent alloy.

As shown by Sockwell et al (1977) amalgams from high copper alloys of the admixture type show up less marginal deterioration than those from their conventional composition counterparts. Starting from two different commercially available conventional composition alloys two different types of admixture alloys were prepared by adding 34 wt.% of a spherical copper containing additive to these conventional powders. One additive was a silver-copper eutectic powder whereas the other one was a ternary Ag (80 wt.%)—Cu (10 wt.%)—Sn (10 wt.%) alloy. Thus in total, four experimental admixture type high copper alloys were obtained. After two years under oral conditions amalgams from all experimental admixture amalgams showed up less marginal breakdown than those from the original conventional alloys. It is interesting to note that no significant differences could be found between amalgams from the four experimental admixture alloys, although amalgams from the alloys with the ternary additive definitely contained $\gamma_2$ phase, (only 70% of the $\gamma_2$ phase was suppressed) whereas the $\gamma_2$ phase could not be detected any more in amalgams from the alloy with the silver-copper eutectic.

On the average, the high copper amalgams show up a better performance than the conventional composition ones with respect to discoloration and roughness of the surface of the restoration. However, there is some overlap in the sense that at least a few amalgams from conventional alloys are more or less equivalent to the high copper amalgams (see e. g. *Letzel* et al., 1977 and 1978a).

Probably, zinc containing conventional amalgams show up better corrosion resistance (apart from delayed expansion) than those prepared from zinc free alloys of the same brand name *(Wilson & Ryge,* 1963). *Leinfelder* et al., (1977) reported as to the influence of burnishing and polishing. The effect of burnishing upon marginal deterioration turned out to be controversial. For an alloy with a relatively short (ultimate) carving time they found that post-carve burnishing resulted in less marginal fracture. Marginal breakdown was not affected by polishing in case of the burnished restoration. *Leinfelder* et al. (1977) described a negative influence of burnishing upon marginal fracture for a slow setting amalgam. Also in this case, polishing of amalgam restorations which had been previously burnished did not improve the situation as to the marginal integrity. For both amalgams, restorations which were not burnished showed up less marginal deterioration in comparison with the not polished ones.

*Letzel* et al. (1978b) found only a slightly significant influence of the factor condensation technic upon roughness and marginal deterioration, whereas no influence could be found with regard to discoloration.

## 3.6. Miscellaneous Properties

As far as the mechanical properties are concerned, in earlier sections, attention has been only given to strength. In text books on dental materials several other properties such as elastic limit, proportional limit, yield strength, hardness, impact strength, ductility, toughness (brittleness), resilience, modulus of elasticitiy, flow and plasticity are dealt with. Furthermore, no attention has been paid to properties such as thermal conductivity, thermal diffusivity, electrical conductivity and linear coefficient of thermal expansion (for a definition of the different terms the reader is referred to text books on (dental) materials science). In this section some remarks will be made as to the importance of these properties.

The modulus of elasticity of both dentin and enamel is small in comparison with that of dental amalgam. This implies, for a certain deformation, stresses to be higher in dental amalgam than in dentin and enamel. This effect is intensified by the fact that the amalgam restoration only replaces part of the tooth structures so that applied forces have to be distributed over a relatively small area. As a result, a narrow isthmus shall not be prepared (see section 3.3.1.2.). However, nothing can be done to lower the modulus of elasticity substantially (unless amalgam could be combined with a resinous material for instance) because its modulus of elasticity is a more or less intrinsic result of its metallic structure. Because the dentist can hardly influence the modulus of elasticity by materials choice or manipulation, no special attention is paid to this property.

Under "normal" service conditions, amalgam should be considered as a brittle material which, due to its relatively low ductility, breaks approximately at the elastic limit (as pointed out by *Philipps* (1973) for practical purposes the terms elastic limit, proportional limit and yield strength can be considered to be synonymous). Due to this low ductility the breaking strength is a good measure for the proportional limit, the elastic limit as well as the yield strength, so that discussion of the latter properties can be omitted.

The modulus of resilience, and thereby the brittleness, probably can be related to the strength of amalgam. However, it must be stressed here that for all different types of amalgam and their manipulation, the material should be considered as brittle in comparison with dentin. This implies small isolated parts of amalgam to be contra-indicated, i. e.: the cavity shall not be bevelled at the occlusal surface, occlusal overhang shall be avoided (see fig. 41) whereas deep carving of fissures cannot be applied. Besides the reasons mentioned in section 3.3.1.2. the brittleness of amalgam is another reason to avoid an extremely thin or shallow isthmus.

Although the hardness test shows up some analogy with the loading conditions in the oral cavity, this measurement is left out of consideration: for short times of loading, hardness is correlated with strength whereas for long times of loading, creep plays a major role as to the outcome of the hardness test.

Flow of the dental amalgam is determined analogously to the creep. Main difference between the two tests is that their respective determinations start at different times. In case of the determination of flow, the load is applied at a time when the material is still hardening (usually 3 hours after trituration), whereas the creep test starts when the amalgam has acquired its full strength (between 1 day and 1 week). Several investigators could not detect any evidence of failure arising from flow (*Sweeney*, 1940; *Phillips* et al., 1945; *Nadal* et al., 1961 a and b; *Mahler,* 1970). Observations on restorations made from amalgams showing up extremely high flow values failed to reveal any evidence of flow, even in case of traumatic occlusion. Thus, this property should be considered as not relevant. However, it might be an appropriate test for the manufacturer to use it during the

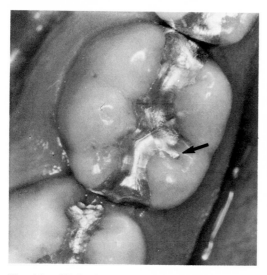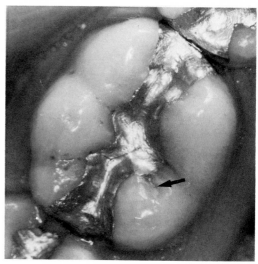

Fig. 41   Clinical case of the fracture of an occlusal overhang.

Fig. 41a   Restoration directly after filling and polishing.

Fig. 41b   Restoration after 6 months; the overhangs already have failed.

manufacturing process as a quality control tool.

Plasticity of the amalgam mix is one of the first properties the dentist is confronted with. A good plasticity is a condition for both an adequate adaptability of the amalgam restoration against the cavity wall and to guarantee an amalgam with a minimum amount of porosities. Although dentists recognize the importance of plasticity hardly any information can be found in dental literature; even a clear definition is lacking. Indeed an obscure situation. Thermal conductivity, thermal diffusivity as well as electrical conductivity are very relevant properties. For example, direct contact of an amalgam restoration with an ice cream might be experienced as a torment. However, the dentist cannot change this situation by means of either the choice of another amalgam alloy or a modified manipulation. Therefore, in case of deep cavities the dentist should anticipate the relatively high thermal conductivity and diffusivity and place a cement base (for a discussion of the effectivity of different base materials see e. g. *Tibbetts* et al., 1976). This cement base has no influence on the current through the pulp. Therefore, in order to minimize the discomfort of initial galvanic shocks an external varnish should be applied on the surface of the amalgam restoration.

### References

*Asgar, K., Arfaei, A. H. & Mahler, D. B.* (1977):
Evaluation of Amalgam Tensile Test Methods.
J. Dent. Res. **56**, Special Issue A, paper 140.

*Bell, G. J.* (1977):
An Elementary Study of Deformation of Molar Teeth During Amalgam Restorative Procedures. Aust. Dent. J. **22**, 177.

Binon, P., Philipps, R. W., Swartz, M. L. Norman, R. D. & Mehra, R. (1973):
Clinical Behaviour of Amalgam as Related to Certain Mechanical Properties. J. Dent. Res. **52,** Special Issue, paper 190.

Charbenau, G. T., Bozell, R. & Carpenter, K. (1977):
Clinical Evaluation of Tytin, Dispersalloy and Spheralloy, J. Dent. Res. **56,** Special Issue A, paper 149.

Darvell, B. W. (1976):
Strength of Dispersalloy Amalgam. Br. Dent. J. **141,** 273.

Dérand, T. (1977):
Marginal Failure of Amalgam Class II Restoration. J. Dent. Res. **56,** 481.

Duperon, D. F., Nevile, M. D. & Kasloff, Z. (1977):
Clinical Evaluation of Corrosion Resistance of Conventional Alloy, Spherical-Particle Alloy, and Dispersion-Phase Alloy. J. Prosthet. Dent. **25,** 650.

Fusayama, T., Katayori, T. & Nomoto, S. (1963):
Corrosion of Gold and Amalgam Placed in Contact with Each Other. J. Dent. Res. **42,** 1183.

Granath, L. E. & Hiltscher, R. (1970):
Strength of Edges of Class II Cavity Restorations in Relation to Buccolingual Shape of Cavity. Odontol. Revy **21,** 189.

Hals, E., Nernaes, A., Simonsen, T. L., Andreassen, B. H., Bie, T., Halse, A., Das, T. K. & Gjerdet, N. R. (1975):
Experimental and Natural Lesions around Silver Amalgam Fillings, in: Proceedings of the International Symposium on Amalgam and Tooth-Coloured Restorative Material. Ed. Van Amerongen, A. J., Dippel, H. W., Spanauf, A. J. & Vrijhoef, M. M. A. Dental School, University of Nijmegen, p. 19.

Jongenburger, P. (1977):
Physical and Phenomenological Models for Creep, in Proceedings International Symposium Prediction of—Residual—Lifetime of Constructions Operating at High Temperature. Netherlands Institute of Welding, The Hague.

Jørgensen, K. D. (1965a):
The Mechanism of Marginal Fracture of Amalgam Fillings. Acta Odontol. Scand. **23,** 347.

Jørgensen, K. D. (1965b):
Adaptability of Dental Amalgam. Acta Odontol. Scand. **23,** 257.

Jørgensen, K. D. & Isenoumi, K. (1969):
The Relationship between Tensile Strength and Carvability of Dental Amalgam. Acta Ondontol. Scand. **27,** 47.

Jørgensen, K. D. (1977):
Amalgame in der Zahnheilkunde. Carl Hanser, München.

Kropp, R., Seyfried, A. & Riethe, P. (1977):
Prüfung verschiedener Methoden zur Bestimmung der Verarbeitungszeit von Amalgam. Dtsch. Zahnärztl. Z. **32,** 871.

Leinfelder, K. F., Sluder, T. B., Strickland, W. D. & Taylor, D. F. (1977):
Two Year Clinical Evaluation of Burnished Amalgam Restorations. J. Dent. Res. **56,** Special Issue B, paper 251.

Letzel, H., Aardening, Ch. J. M. W., Fick, J. M. & Vrijhoef, M. M. A. (1977):
Marginal Breakdown of Amalgam Restorations versus Creep. J. Dent. Res. **56,** Special Issue A, paper 245.

Letzel, H., Aardening, Ch. J. M. M., Fick, J. M., Van Leusen, J. & Vrijhoef, M. M. A. (1978a):
Tarnish, Corrosion and Marginal Fracture of Amalgam Restorations. J. Dent. Res. **57,** Special Issue A, paper 356.

Letzel, H., Aardening, Ch. J. M. W., Fick, J. M., Van Leusen, J. & Vrijhoef, M. M. A. (1978b):
Condensation Technic versus Clinical Behavior of Amalgam Restorations. J. Dent. Res. **57,** Special Issue A, paper 497.

Mahler, D. B. (1958):
An Analysis of Stresses in a Dental Amalgam Restoration. J. Dent. Res. **37,** 516.

Mahler, D. B., Terkla, L. G., Van Eysden, J. & Reisbick, M. H. (1970):
Marginal Fracture versus Mechanical Properties of Amalgam. J. Dent. Res. **49,** 1452.

Mahler, D. B., Terkla, L. G. & Van Eysden, J. (1973):
Marginal Fracture of Amalgam Restorations. J. Dent. Res. **52,** 823.

Mahler, D. B., Van Eysden, J. & Terkla, L. G. (1975):
Relationship of Creep to Marginal Fracture of Amalgam. J. Dent. Res. **54,** Special Issue A, paper 553.

*Marxkors, R.* (1970):
Korrosionserscheinungen an Amalgamfül-lungen und deren Auswirkungen auf den menschlichen Organismus, Teil II. Dtsch. Zahnärztl. Z. **24**, 117.

*Mathewson, R. J., Brunner, F. W. & Noonan, R. G.* (1967):
The Clinical Comparison of a Spherical Amal-gam Alloy and a Conventional Amalgam Alloy: A Pilot Study. J. Dent. Child. **34**, 176.

*Mathewson, R. J., Retzlaff, A. E. & Porter, D. R.* (1973):
Marginal Failure of Amalgam Restorations in Primary Teeth Related to Material Selection and Proximal Retention. J. Prosthet. Dent. **29**, 288.

*Mathewson, R. J., Retzlaff, A. E. & Porter, D. R.* (1974):
Marginal Failure in Deciduous Teeth: A Two-Year Report. J. Am. Dent. Assoc. **88**, 134.

*Moffa, J. P. & Jenkins, W. A.* (1977):
Two Year Clinical Evaluation of a Dispersed Phase and a Single Phase Amalgam. J. Dent. Res. **56**, Special Issue B, paper 248.

*Mumford, J. M.* (1960):
Pain Due to Galvanism. Br. Dent. J. **108**, 299.

*Nachlin, J. J.* (1954):
A Type of Pain Associated with the Restora-tion of Teeth with Amalgam. J. Am. Dent. Assoc. **48**, 284.

*Nadal, R., Phillips, R. W. & Swartz, M. L.* (1961a):
Clinical Investigation on the Relation of Mer-cury to the Amalgam Restoration: I J. Am. Dent. Assoc. **63**, 8.

*Nadal, R., Phillips, R. W. & Swartz, M. L.* (1961b):
Clinical Investigation on the Relation of Mercury to the Amalgam Restoration: II J. Am. Dent. Assoc. **63**, 488.

*Ohashi, M., Ware, A. L. & Docking, A. R.* (1975):
A Comparison of Methods for Determining Setting Rate of Amalgam. Aust. Dent. J. **20**, 176.

*Osborne, J. W. & Gale, E. N.* (1974a):
Long Term Follow-up of Clinical Evaluations of Lathe-Cut versus Spherical Amalgam. J. Dent, Res. **53**, 1204.

*Osborne, J. W. & Gale, E. N.* (1974b):
A Two-, Three-, and Four Year Follow-up of a Clinical Study of the Effect of Trituration on Amalgam Restorations. J. Am. Dent. Assoc. **88**, 795.

*Osborne, J. W., Phillips, R. W., Gale, E. N. & Binon, P. P.* (1976):
Three-Year Clinical Comparison of Three Amalgam Alloy Types Emphasizing an Apprai-sal of the Evaluation Methods Used. J. Am. Dent. Assoc. **93**, 784.

*Osborne, J. W., Phillips, R. W., Swartz, M. L. & Norman, R. D.* (1977a):
Influence of Certain Manipulative Variables on the Static Creep of Amalgam. J. Dent. Res. **56**, 616.

*Osborne, J. W., Swartz, M. L., Gale, E. N. & Phillips, R. W.* (1977b):
Clinical Performance of Ten Amalgam Alloys. A One-Year Report. J. Dent. Res. **56**, Special Issue B, paper 250.

*Osborne, J. W., Gale, E. N., Coch, D. & Phillips, R. W.* (1978):
Clinical Assessment of Marginal Breakdown of Nine High Copper Content Amalgams. J. Dent. Res. **57**, Special Issue A, paper 26.

*Phillips, R. W., Boyd, D. A., Healy, H. J. & Crawford, W. N.* (1945):
Clinical Observations on Amalgam with Known Physical Properties, Final Report. J. Am. Dent. Assoc. **32**, 325.

*Phillips, R. W.* (1957):
Die Bedeutung elektrischer Ströme in der Mundhöhle. Dtsch. Zahnärztl. Z. **12**, 1222.

*Phillips, R. W., Gilmore, H. W., Swartz, M. L. & Schenker, S. I.* (1961):
Adaptation of Restorations in Vivo as Asses-sed by $Ca^{45}$. J. Am. Dent. Assoc. **62**, 9.

*Phillips, R. W.* (1973):
Skinner's Science of Dental Materials, 7th Ed., W. B. Saunders, Philadelphia.

*Powell, G. L., Nicholls, J. I. & Shurtz, D. E.* (1977):
Deformation of Human Teeth under the Action of an Amalgam Matrix Band. Oper. Dentistry, **2**, 64.

*Rupp, N. W., Pfaffenbarger, G. C. & Manuszewski, R. C.* (1977):
Amalgam Restoration: Part I, Margin Integrity. J. Dent. Res. **56**, Special Issue A, paper 242.

*Schoonover, T. C. & Souder, W.* (1941):
Corrosion of Dental Alloys, J. Am. Dent. Assoc. **28**, 1278.

Sockwell, C. L., Leinfelder, K. F. & Taylor, D. F. (1977):
Two-Year Clinical Evaluation of Experimental Copper Additive Amalgams. J. Dent. Res. **56**, Special Issue B, paper 249.

Spanauf, A. J., Vermeersch, A. G. & Vrijhoef, M. M. A. (1976a):
La Résistance aux Forces de Tractions de l'Amalgame Après 15 Minutes. Rev. Belge Méd. Dent. **31**, 225.

Spanauf, A. J., Vermeersch, A. G. & Vrijhoef, M. M. A. (1976b):
La Résistance aux Forces de Tractions de Differentes Marques d'Amalgame. Rev. Belge Méd. Dent. **31**, 341.

Spanauf, A. J. (1977):
Manipulative Techniques versus Dimensional Change, Creep and Strength of Different Amalgams. Thesis, Nijmegen.

Spanauf, A. J., Vrijhoef, M. M. A. & De Graaf, R. (1977a):
The Influence of Some Manipulative Factors on Creep. Aust. Dent. J. **22**, 203.

Spanauf, A. J., Vrijhoef, M. M. A. & De Graaf, R. (1977b):
The Influence of the Dentist upon Dimensional Change and Creep of Amalgam. Aust. Dent. J. **22**, 351.

Sweeney, J. T. (1940):
Amalgam Manipulation: Manual vs. Mechanical Aids. Part II: Comparison of Clinical Applications. J. Am. Dent. Assoc. **27**, 1940.

Tibbetts, V. R., Schnell, R. J., Swartz, M. L. & Phillips, R. W. (1976):
Thermal Diffusion through Amalgam and Cement Bases: Comparison of in Vitro and in Vivo Measurements. J. Dent. Res. **55**, 441.

Vermeersch, A. G. (1975):
Restaurations d'Hemi-Arcades à l'Amalgame. Rev. Belge. Méd. Dent. **30**, 377.

Vrijhoef, M. M. A. (1973):
Dental Amalgam. An Explorative Study. Thesis, Nijmegen.

Vrijhoef, M. M. A., Spanauf, A. J. & Driessens, F. C. M. (1975):
Execessive Long-Term Dimensional Change of Amalgam. Aust. Dent. J. **20**, 37.

Vrijhoef, M. M. A. (1975):
On the Improvement of the Life-Time of Amalgam Restorations, in: Proceedings of the International Symposium on Amalgam and Tooth-Coloured Restorative Material. Ed. Van Amerongen, A. J., Dippel, H. W., Spanauf, A. J. & Vrijhoef, M. M. A. Dental School, University of Nijmegen, p. 37.

Vrijhoef, M. M. A., Vermeersch, A. G. & Spanauf, A. J. (1979):
Diametral Tensile Strength of 23 Hardened Commercial Amalgams. J. Oral Rehabil. **6**, 153.

Watson, P. A., Phillips, R. W., Swartz, M. L. & Gilmore, H. W. (1973):
A Comparison of Zinc-Containing and Zinc-Free Amalgam Restorations. J. Prosthet. Dent. **29**, 536.

Weaver, R. G., Johnson, B. E., McCune, R. J. & Cvar, J. F. (1970):
Three-Year Clinical Evaluation of a Spherical Dental Amalgam Alloy. IADR/NAD, New York, DMG Microfilm, paper 267.

Wilson, C. J. & Ryge, G. (1963):
Clinical Study of Dental Amalgam. J. Am. Dent. Assoc. **66**, 763.

# 4. Chemical Composition and Microstructure of Amalgam Versus Properties

## 4.1. Introduction

Properties of a material are dependent upon composition and microstructure. In case of dental amalgam both the manufacturer and the dental team contribute to the ultimate chemical composition, the microstructure, the properties as well as the behavior of amalgam restorations under oral conditions. Concerning the behavior of the amalgam restoration in the oral cavity the patient has got the last word.

In this chapter attention will be mainly paid to the contribution of the factor dentist. It will be dealt more or less explicitly with the factor manufacturer if the differences between the respective commercial amalgams are significant under oral conditions.

In section 4.2 some attention will be given to microstructural aspects being important to most properties discussed so far. In section 4.3 it will be dealt at length with relations between on the one hand properties and on the other hand chemical composition as well as microstructure. Finally, in section 4.4 the influence of the dental team upon chemical composition and microstructure will be dealt with. This section is very important because a substantial part of the failures of amalgam restorations are due to manipulative errors. Trends thus deduced from the latter section can be used either to predict or to explain the influence of the dental team upon the properties of dental amalgam and thereby upon the performance of amalgam restorations under oral conditions. These last aspects will be dealt with at length in chapter 5.

## 4.2. Microstructure of Amalgam

As might be deduced from section 2.5 the phase composition of the different commercial amalgams varies considerably. Factors related to the production, such as chemical composition, melting technic, the different heat treatments and the manipulation by the dental team influence the microstructure of the amalgam substantially. In spite of these important influences, for most purposes the microstructure of a dental amalgam can be adequately described as a composite material whereby the remnants of the original alloy particles are embedded in a matrix of the newly formed reaction products (see chapter 2). It is obvious that, once the amalgam alloy has been chosen, the residual mercury content plays a major role. As for a certain commercial amalgam, this relation is shown in fig. 42. It is characteristic for the available commercial

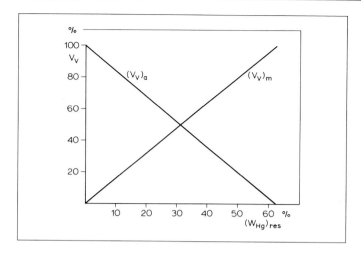

Fig. 42 Dependence of the amount of both alloy particles $(V_v)_a$ and matrix phases $(V_v)_m$ upon the residual mercury content for a particular conventional composition amalgam (computed from Vrijhoef & Driessens, 1974a).

amalgams that the original alloy particles disappear completely at a residual mercury content of 60–70 wt.%. In case of high copper amalgams generally the matrix phases contain only a minute amount of $\gamma_2$ phase (a few tenths of a percent by volume). However, some commercial high copper amalgams contain a substantial amount of $\gamma_2$ phase, and at most can be considered as $\gamma_2$-reduced. It must be stressed here that the remaining non-$\gamma_2$ amalgams cannot be considered to be $\gamma_2$-free apart from a few tenths of a percent under all circumstances; mainly due to the residual mercury content which plays an important role. Above a certain critical limit these amalgams contain $\gamma_2$ phase *(Jensen, 1977; Malhotra & Asgar, 1978)*. This critical mercury level is given in table 4 for some commercial high copper amalgams (see also fig. 43).

In chapter 2 it has been stressed that porosity is more or less an intrinsic feature of dental amalgam. By means of the parameters of the manufacturing process of the amalgam alloy, such as particle size and heat treatments, the porosity content of the resulting amalgam can be partially controlled. An example is given in fig. 44.

The manufacturer attempts a minimization of this type of porosity. For the different certified commercial amalgams the maximum amount of this type of porosity is of the order of one percent by volume or less (see e. g. *Espevik, 1977c*). In the following parts of this chapter this type of porosity will be omitted.

Table 4
Lowest mercury content at which $\gamma_2$ phase occurs in some commercial high copper amalgams.

| Aristalloy CR | 44 |
|---|---|
| Cupraloy | > 60 |
| Dispersalloy | > 60 |
| Indiloy | 49 |
| Luxalloy | > 60 |
| Micro II | < 35 |
| Optalloy II | < 35 |
| Sybraloy | > 60 |
| Tytin | 47 |

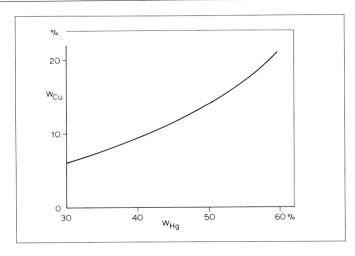

Fig. 43 Critical mercury limit for a hypothetical all-in-one alloy system. Above this limit $\gamma_2$ phase occurs in the amalgam. Computed on the basis that the amalgam consists of $Ag_3Sn$ plus $Cu_3Sn$, whereby it has been assumed that all $Cu_3Sn$ reacts with Sn to form $Cu_6Sn_5$.

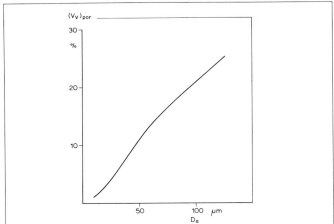

Fig. 44 The dependence of the porosity content of an amalgam made from a silver (74%)-tin (26%) alloy upon the particle size of the amalgam alloy (adapted from Taylor, 1972).

However, it must be stressed here that careless production of the amalgam alloy leads to an excessive porosity content of the amalgam and therefore jeopardizes its properties. Other factors determining the porosity content of the amalgam are related to its manipulation. These factors will be discussed in section 4.4.

## 4.3. Residual Mercury Content and Microstructure Versus Properties

### 4.3.1. Strength

Four typical examples of the dependence of the compressive strength upon the residual mercury content are given in fig. 45.
It might be concluded that in all cases compressive strength decreases with increasing residual mercury content. A

1% increase of the residual mercury content corresponds with a decrease of the compressive strength of 5—11 $MN/m^2$. On a relative scale this causes a 1% loss of compressive strength per 1% increase of the residual mercury content*. These data are consistent with those reported by *Jørgensen, Esbensen & Borring-Møller* (1966). *Mahler & Mitchem* (1964) reported much higher values. This might be due to the fact that the porosity content was not adequately controlled in their experiments. According to *Jørgensen* et al. (1966) an increase of the porosity with one percent by volume corresponds with a ten percent decrease of the strength approximately. Thus an adequate control of the porosity is extremely important. Up to now, no systematic simultaneous description of the influence of both residual mercury content and amount of porosity upon the strength of commercial dental amalgams has been reported. Therefore, no information is available as to the interaction effects of mercury and porosity content. Another important factor determining the strength of a multiphase material such as dental amalgam, is the quality of the bond between the original alloy particles and the matrix phases. Several investigators *(Young & Wilsdorf,* 1972; *Darvell,* 1976) showed that the removal of an oxide layer from the dental amalgam alloy particles substantially improves the bond between these particles and the newly formed matrix phases, and therefore leads to a higher strength. As shown by *Young & Wilsdorf* (1972), the experimental scatter of

the strength data is positively influenced by such a treatment as well. This effect has been described both for conventional composition amalgams *(Young & Wilsdorf,* 1972) and high copper ones of the admixture type *(Darvell,* 1976). In the latter case, atmospheric oxidation of the silver-copper particles not only gives an inferior bond between these particles and the newly formed matrix phases, but also results in a less efficient suppression of the $\gamma_2$ phase. Next to the residual mercury content the influence of the porosity content is extremely important.

At present, the fracture mechanism of dental amalgam has not been completely elucidated. However, it is reasonable to assume that the fracture mechanism of conventional composition amalgams is controlled by the separation of the matrix phases. In case of high copper amalgams both separation and cleavage of the $\gamma_1$ phase play a role *(Okabe* et al., 1977). This might explain the observed higher strength values for some high copper amalgams.

### 4.3.2. Dimensional change

#### 4.3.2.1. Setting changes

Dimensional change during hardening depends on several factors. Primarily, dimensional changes during hardening of dental amalgams can be explained on the basis of (a) the elimination of pores existing after trituration, (b) the introduction of empty spaces due to mass transport in the setting amalgam, as well as (c) on the basis of the difference between on the one hand the mean specific gravity of the initial alloy

---

* The same trend is found for (diametral) tensile strength, although a larger scatter of the data makes the result statistically less significant.

Fig. 45 a

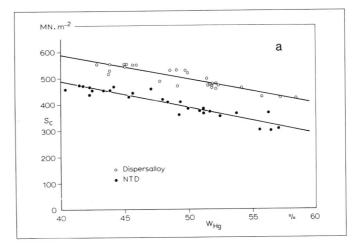

Fig. 45 b

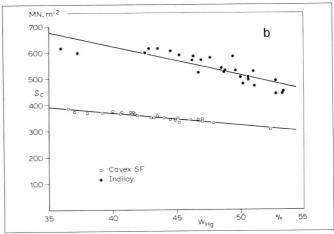

Fig. 45 Four examples of the dependence of the compressive strength upon the residual mercury content: (a) New True Dentalloy (conventional composition, lathe cut) and Dispersalloy (high copper, admixture type). (b) Cavex SF (conventional composition, spherical) and Indiloy (high copper, spherical all-in-one).

powder plus mercury and on the other hand that of the phases of the set amalgam. It is obvious that the mechanism described under (a) leads to a contraction, whereas (b) gives rise to an expansion. The contribution due to the specific gravity difference referred to under (c) strongly depends upon the initial chemical composition and microstructure of the amalgam alloy as well as upon the residual mercury content and the resulting phase composition of the corresponding amalgam. However, in case of most commercial amalgams it gives either a very slight contraction or expansion within the range ±20 µm/cm. A fourth factor, being extremely important for the actual dimensional change during setting, is the state of the amalgam mix at the time when it is adapted against the cavity wall. For example, phase changes which have been realized before the amalgam was brought into the cavity cannot contribute any more to the dimensional change occurring in the cavity. One of the most important factors controlling the dimensional change during hardening is the residual mercury content. As might be judged from fig. 22 the influence of the residual mercury content is of special interest for percentages larger than 55 wt.% approximately. Above this mercury level, the hardening expansion increases dramatically with increasing mercury content and gives unacceptable clinical results. Note that the time of observation is very important and wholly or partially determines the conclusion from the experiment.

This time dependence can be easily understood on the basis of the fact that these dimensional changes can be correlated with the rate of solid-solid phase transformations which occur at a much lower rate than the initial setting reactions in which liquid mercury is involved. Because no information is available as to the different commercial products no definite conclusions can be drawn. However, on the basis of the work reported by *Jørgensen, Christiansen & Esbensen* (1973) it is plausible to assume that this effect might be generalized for the other products as well. They investigated the extra (mercuroscopic) expansion in case if extra mercury was added. Some examples of their results are given in table 5.

The manufacturer can influence the dimensional change during hardening by means of factors such as chemical composition, average particle size, particle size distribution and heat treatments. An example is given in fig. 46. The manufacturer mainly influences the importance of the solution hardening mechanism relative to the precipitation type of setting. As the dimensional change during setting of the certified amalgams is situated in the region

Table 5
Mercuroscopic expansion at 37° C after 70 days for some commercially available dental amalgams (according to *Jørgensen* et al., 1973).

| Alloy | Expansion (%)<br>$\bar{x}$ (sd) |
|---|---|
| 1 | 5.64 (0.31) |
| 2 | 5.59 (0.36) |
| 3 | 5.34 (0.22) |
| 4 | 5.60 (0.28) |
| 5 | 5.91 (0.17) |

$- 20$ µm/cm to $+ 20$ µm/cm, which is of no clinical significance, no attention will be given to the factor manufacturer.

### 4.3.2.2. Delayed expansion

From chapter 3 it is obvious that necessary conditions for the occurrence of delayed expansion are the contamination of the amalgam mix with water as well as the presence of zinc in the amalgam. Collection of hydrogen, one of the products of the occurring "internal" corrosion, in the amalgam results in an internal pressure, causing an excessive expansion. Probably, creep is the process relaxing the internal stress. Although no systematic research is available, there are indications that the delayed expansion is smaller for amalgams, showing up less creep (see e. g. *Eames, Tharp & Hubbard,* 1973). The amount of delayed expansion is directly related to the amount of contamination so that more contamination gives more delayed expansion. For example, a small amount of contamination caused by perspiration gives less delayed expansion than a lot of contamination due to the presence of saliva in the cavity (*Jørgensen,* 1977).

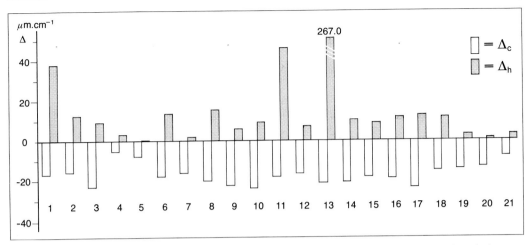

Fig. 46    The influence of an additional heat treatment at 435°C on the dimensional change during hardening.
$\Delta_c$: alloys in the "as received" condition; $\Delta_h$: alloys after an additional heat treatment at 435°C (according to Vrijhoef & Driessens, 1975c).

Water always condenses on parts of the instruments such as the condensing points because the relative low temperature of these instruments is lower than the dew point in the oral cavity. This water only gives a very slight delayed expansion, which probably has no clinical significance (Jørgensen, 1977). Similarly, a moderate amount of water, which is always present at the wall of a carefully dried cavity is not fatal as for the success of the restoration.

### 4.3.3. Creep

Although the mechanism of creep has not been completely elucidated at present it is clear that the creep of the amalgam is mainly determined by the creep properties of the matrix of reaction products (Vrijhoef & Driessens, 1974b; Espevik, 1977a). The manufacturer might contribute substantially to the creep resistance of the resulting amalgam. Although extensive and detailed investigations are lacking the following remarks can be made. In an investigation comprising commercial conventional composition amalgams Vrijhoef & Jensen (1977) showed the influence of the chemical composition, particle form and heat treatment of the alloy powder to be significant. Amalgams from spherical alloys (other factors being kept constant!) show up less creep than from conventional ones, which may be explained on the basis of a dislocation model. An increase of the zinc content gives less creep. It turned out that the temperature of the heat treatment has an enormous influence (Vrijhoef & Jensen, 1977), which underlines the important and delicate role of the manufacturer. As to the influence of the manufacturer upon the creep of high copper amalgams, the manufacturer plays an equally significant role. For example, fig. 47 shows the

73

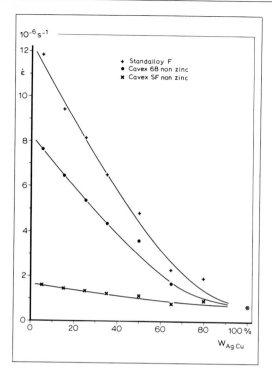

Fig. 47 The creep rate as a function of the silver-copper eutectic content for three different high copper alloys of the admixture type which have been produced from three commercial conventional composition alloys (according to Vrijhoef & Driessens, 1975b, by permission of the Editor of the Journal of Oral Rehabilitation).

influence of the silver-copper eutectic content of three different experimental admixture type alloys upon the creep of the corresponding amalgams *(Vrijhoef & Driessens, (1975b)*. The three experimental admixture type alloys were obtained by mixing silver-copper eutectic alloy with three different, commercially available, dental amalgam alloys. From fig. 47 it may be concluded that the creep resistance of an amalgam prepared from an admixture type amalgam alloy is mainly controlled by the choice of both the (original) amalgam alloy and by the ratio of this alloy to the eutectic alloy.

The relatively improved creep resistance of the high copper amalgams might be explained by the presence of finely dispersed $Cu_6Sn_5$ particles in the

$\gamma_1$ matrix. These $Cu_6Sn_5$ particles are assumed to act as obstacles for the movement of dislocations and thereby improve the creep resistance (Okabe et al., 1977). At this moment, the relation between creep and microstructure is little elucidated.

Up to now, no correlation could be found between the phase composition of dental amalgam and creep *(Mahler & Adey, 1977)*. *Mahler & Adey* (1977) showed that the grain size of the $\gamma_1$ phase plays an important role, whereas the size of the original alloy particles turned out to be important as well. They reported that a finer grain size of the $\gamma_1$ and $\gamma$ particles gives more creep. No significant influence of either the size or the volume of the $\gamma_2$ phase could be established *(Mahler & Adey, 1977)*.

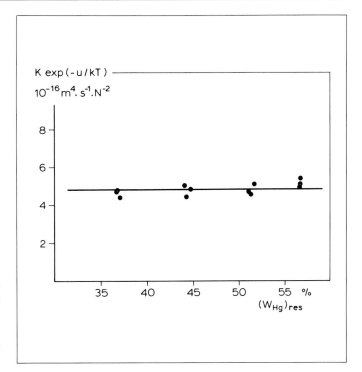

Fig. 48 The dependence of K exp (–U/kT) for a particular amalgam (see equation (4.1) upon the residual mercury content (data from Vrijhoef & Driessens, 1974b).

As reported by *Vrijhoef & Driessens* (1974b), the steady-state creep rate of dental amalgam under the influence of compressive stresses can be described by the formula

$$\dot{\varepsilon} = K (\sigma - \sigma_0)^2 \exp (-U/kT) \qquad (4.1)$$

where $\dot{\varepsilon}$ is the steady-state creep rate, $\sigma$ is the applied stress, $\sigma_0$ is an internal stress component opposing the externally applied stress, U is the activation energy, T is the temperature measured in the Kelvin scale[*], k is the Boltzmann constant and K is a constant of the material.

At a constant temperature the term K exp (–U/kT) turned out to be strongly dependent upon the choice of the amalgam alloy. However, within the errors of

the experiment, it is independent of the residual amount of mercury (see fig. 48). From formula (4.1) it is evident that the steady-state creep rate depends dramatically upon the test temperature. Fig. 49 manifests this influence. $\sigma_0$ which is the order of 10 MN/m$^2$ or less, decreases slightly with increasing temperature and increasing mercury content. The dependence of the steady-state creep rate upon the residual mercury content (see fig. 37) might be explained on the basis of the dependence of $\sigma_0$ upon the mercury content. The dramatic dependence of the creep upon the residual mercury content above a certain critical level has been reported for both conventional composition amalgams (*Vrijhoef & Driessens*, 1974b; *Jørgensen*, 1975; *Mahler*,

---

[*] the zero of the Kelvin scale corresponds roughly to –273°C

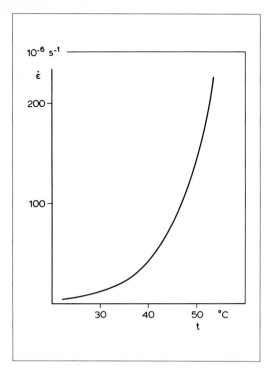

Fig. 49 The influence of the test temperature upon the creep rate of a particular amalgam (computed from equation (4.1) on the basis of Vrijhoef & Driessens, 1974b).

*Adey & Marantz,* 1978) and high copper amalgams *(Mahler* et al., 1978).

Creep increases with increasing porosity content. *Jørgensen* (1975) reported porosity to have a substantial effect upon creep. Increase of the porosity content with one percent by volume affects the creep with 30 percent approximately. It is not known whether this finding holds true for high copper amalgam systems as well. Probably, the interaction of the porosity content with the amount of residual mercury is of importance as well.

As mentioned before (cf. chapter 2) solid-solid transformations occur in the dental amalgams for periods in the order of one year. Due to these phase changes creep depends upon the annealing time at 37°C as well. Although the creep changes vary from amalgam to amalgam, the ranking of the different amalgams remains unchanged *(Vrijhoef & Driessens,* 1975a; *Espevik,* 1977b). Some examples are given in fig. 50.

### 4.3.4. Corrosion

The microstructure of dental amalgam is non-homogeneous by nature: remnants of the alloy particles being embedded in a matrix of reaction products. The corrosion resistance of such a multiphase structure depends on both the intrinsic corrosion properties of the respective phases and microstructural features such as particle size and degree of contiguity of these phases. However, corrosion is not an au-

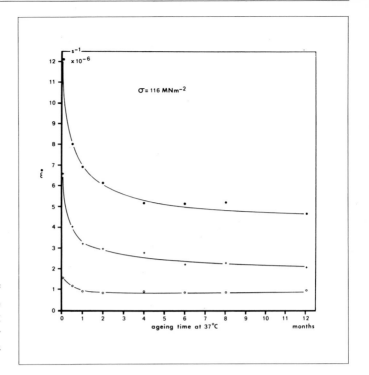

Fig. 50 The dependence of the steady-state creep rate on ageing the amalgam at 37°C for three different amalgams (according to Vrijhoef & Driessens, 1975a).

tonomous process because it is strongly dependent upon the electrochemical interaction between the amalgam and the environment. This may be part of the explanation why no satisfactory predictive corrosion test is available. Although corrosion tests carried out in the laboratory have enhanced our knowledge as to the actual mechanisms of the corrosion of dental amalgam, all different aspects of corrosion cannot be predicted by one parameter of a particular corrosion test. Therefore a combination of different tests is necessary (anodic polarization, corrosion current, corrosion potential, weight change, . . .). Unfortunately, it is difficult to simulate the oral environment in a simple laboratory experiment. However, there are some facts which can be written

about the influence of the microstructure upon the corrosion behavior. As far as conventional composition amalgams are concerned, it is an established fact that the $\gamma_2$ phase is the weakest link. This is obvious from both laboratory experiments and clinical investigations. Depending upon the diet of the patient, corrosion products of tin in the form of oxides, sulfides or chlorides have been reported (see e. g. *Mateer & Reitz,* 1970; *Otani, Jesser & Wilsdorf,* 1973; *Holland & Asgar,* 1974; *Sarkar* et al., 1975). Apparently oxides are always present. These corrosion products might leach out of the restoration and fill up the interspace between the amalgam restoration and the cavity wall. Diffusion into the dentine is possible as well, causing a discoloration of the dentine which can be clinically observed (see e.g. *Hals* et al., 1975).

Mercury does not take part in the electrochemical processes. Mercury which is liberated during the corrosion of the $\gamma_2$ phase remains in the restoration and reacts with the remnants of the alloy particles rather than diffusing into the adjacent biologic tissues. Consequently, *Hals* et al. (1975) could not find mercury in the dentine next to an amalgam restoration. This absence of mercury or corrosion products of mercury in the biological tissues, indicating that the liberated mercury stays in the restoration, may explain why no major adverse effects are known with respect to dental amalgam. Because of the corrosion of the $\gamma_2$ phase, once a certain conventional amalgam alloy has been chosen, it is a wise policy to reduce the amount of $\gamma_2$ phase as much as possible. As shown in section 4.2 the amount of $\gamma_2$ phase is proportional to the residual mercury content. From the work of *Nadal, Phillips & Swartz* (1961) it is obvious that an amalgam restoration with a higher mercury content gives a rougher surface and more marginal breakdown after functioning for a certain time under oral conditions. On a laboratory scale, *Jørgensen* (1972) nicely demonstrated the influence of the corrosion of the $\gamma_2$ phase upon the strength. He reported that an increase of the $\gamma_2$ content corresponding with a 1% increase of the residual mercury content gives a 1% loss of diametral tensile strength after corrosion. *Averette, Hochman & Marek* (1978) reported up to 50% loss of compressive strength for conventional composition amalgams. For the high copper amalgams they found some loss of strength as well (on the average 11%; substantial differences between the respective amalgams).

Care should be taken in case of comparing two different dental amalgams. It is not necessarily true that the amalgam with the least amount of $\gamma_2$ phase shows up less detrimental effects due to corrosion. If one compares two different conventional composition amalgams the distribution of the $\gamma_2$ phase plays a role as well. If the $\gamma_2$ phase tends to appear as isolated particles in the matrix the amalgam will show up less corrosion, even if more $\gamma_2$ phase is present. In section 3.5.2 it was shown that marginal deterioration problems are not necessarily solved if the $\gamma_2$ content is either reduced or eliminated. In case if no $\gamma_2$ phase is present at all there is still corrosion. Although there is some contradictory data given about this subject it is reasonable to assume that the $Cu_6Sn_5$ is the phase most prone to corrosion in non-$\gamma_2$ amalgams *(Marek & Okabe, 1977)*. In some high copper amalgams (in vitro) loss of copper was observed during corrosion *(Averette* et al., 1978) Its clinical relevance is still unknown.

As might be judged from table 4 several high copper amalgams contain the $\gamma_2$ phase at a moderate or high mercury content. At this time, the consequences of the presence of considerable amounts of the $\gamma_2$ phase in high copper amalgams is unknown. It is obvious that the corrosion resistance strongly depends upon the amount of porosity. As reported by *Jørgensen* (1975) the influence of a 1–2% increase of the porosity content upon the corrosion is of the same order as the differences between the respective commercial conventional composition amalgams.

### 4.3.5. Adaptability

It is obvious that a relatively high mercury content gives good rheologic properties and thereby contributes to a superior adaptation against the cavity wall. It must be stressed here that the term "high mercury content" strongly depends upon the choice of the amalgam alloy. For example, in case of some spherical alloys acceptable results can be obtained with 45 wt.% mercury, or even less, whereas some of the traditional lathe cut alloys demand more than 55 wt.% to attain a reasonable adaptability. As discussed in the previous sections, a high residual mercury content is detrimental to most of the properties. Therefore, a high initial mercury content should be reduced either before or during packing. The fact that porosity at the amalgam surface adjacent to the cavity wall jeopardizes an acceptable adaptability needs no further explanation.

## 4.4. Manipulation Versus Chemical Composition and Microstructure

### 4.4.1. Choice of factors

Before the restoration of the teeth is undertaken, the dentist is forced to take a substantial number of decisions. First of all, the alloy to be used should be selected. If we assume the dental practitioner to make his or her choice from the amalgam alloys certified by the American Dental Association, there are 150 alternatives approximately, comprising both conventional composition and high copper alloys, zinc- or non-zinc preparations, course-, fine- or micro-grain alloys, pre-amalgamated or without

mercury, spherical or lathe-cut alloys. Generally, each of these 150 alloys can be delivered either in the powder form (in bulk or pre-capsulated) or as pellets. Trituration can be done by means of at least 20 different amalgamators. Once the choice is made for hand packing or condensation by means of a mechanical vibrator, within each type ten different possibilities are available at least. In order not to give the impression that the problem is exaggerated by us only ten different combinations of carving and polishing are assumed to be available, including a choice from the different instruments and materials available. If the number of alternatives to be chosen from is based upon the figures mentioned, the dentist can make his choice from 150 x 3 x 20 x 2 x 10 x 10 = 1,800,000 different modes of manipulation. The dental materials scientist has even to deal with more factors such as trituration time, delay between trituration and condensation, packing forces, etc., etc. It is obvious that a profound and systematic investigation of all available combinations is impossible. Therefore, it will be resticted to the most important features. The trends deduced from their influence upon chemical composition and microstructure form the framework from which the influence of other treatment combinations can be predicted. The qualitative character of the matter will be reinforced by the omission of the dimension of properties in the different figures of this section.

### 4.4.2. Initial mercury content

As given in fig. 51 residual mercury content increases with increasing initial amount of mercury (other factors kept

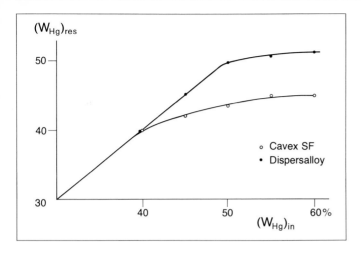

Fig. 51 Influence of the initial mercury content upon the residual amount of mercury.

constant!). Thus, the residual mercury content might be reduced by minimizing the initial mercury content.

This technic is referred to as the Eames or dry-mix technic *(Eames,* 1959). It is feasible that the initial mercury content can be reduced as long as the plasticity remains acceptable. In general, this technic is a suitable one for modern amalgam alloys, especially in case of major part of the spherical alloys, showing up a superior plasticity. For a part of the older types lathe-cut alloys this technic cannot be applied. Major part of the already available alloys before the second world war showed relatively bad wettability of the alloy particles with mercury. In these cases the mercury content could be reduced by squeezing the wet amalgam mix in a linen cloth before condensation has been commenced (see e. g. *Sweeney & Burns,* 1961). If a high mercury content is present during condensation special care shall be taken so as to express a sufficient amount of mercury during packing (see section 4.4.5). Disadvantage of the "wet" technics is that much

more amalgam alloy and mercury is used (see e. g. *Bergdahl,* 1973).

In case if an adequate, controlled, technic is used such as advocated by *Jørgensen* (1977) the amount of porosity decreases with increasing initial mercury content, as represented schematically in fig. 52.

Characteristic for this dependence is that the porosity content is independent of the initial amount of mercury for mercury percentages above a certain value. This value depends strongly upon the choice of the amalgam alloy. The relation given in fig. 52 can be easily understood on the basis of the fact that a minimum plasticity is necessary in order to make it possible to reduce the porosity content below an acceptable level. Generally, spherical alloys give a good plasticity at a relatively low initial mercury content. In these cases the critical mercury content given in fig. 52 is 45 wt.% approximately or even lower. The minimum amount of porosity in fig. 52 corresponds with the porosity intrinsically formed during hardening. As shown in section 2.6 this amount of

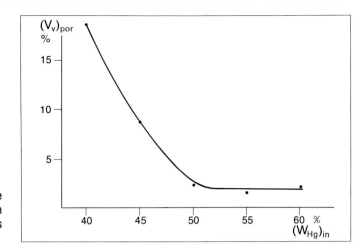

Fig. 52 Influence of the initial mercury content upon the amount of porosities present in the set amalgam.

### 4.4.3. Triduration

One of the main objectives of trituration is to obtain a thorough, homogeneous mixture of amalgam alloy and mercury. During mixing the setting reactions are initiated. In case if the mixing is not too vigorously carried out, porosities will be removed from the plastic amalgam mix. In case of a relatively long trituration time, the plasticitiy of the amalgam mass will become inferior, already formed reaction products will be broken up, condensation cannot be carried out effectively any more, and, consequently, porosity content will increase with increasing trituration time. A schematic representation of the influence of the mixing time upon the amount of porosity is given in fig. 53.

The rationale of this figure are the processes occurring during trituration. As shown in fig. 54a the trituration time does not influence the residual mercury content in case of New True Dentalloy. This example holds true for many conventional composition lathe cut alloys. It illustrates that wetting the alloy with mercury is predominant at this stage rather than a genuine hardening reaction with the latter. Cavex SF shows quite another dependence. Initially the trituration time does not influence the residual mercury content. Then the residual mercury content increases with increasing trituration time. At a certain trituration time the graph shows up a steep negative slope. This dependence might be explained as follows. Probably, mercury penetrates between the grains of the alloy particles (see fig. 14d) and remains there in a liquid state. The mercury which penetrated along the grain boundaries cannot be any more removed during condensation. Therefore, the residual mercury content increases with increasing trituration time.

Due to the penetration of the mercury into the alloy particles, the bonding between the grains of one alloy particle

porosity which is 1% by volume or less, cannot be reduced by means of a careful manipulation.

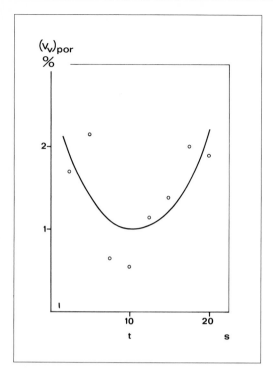

Fig. 53 Dependence of the porosity content upon the trituration time.

is weakened. The alloy particles are broken up at a certain critical trituration time. As a result, more mercury becomes available which can be removed during condensation and the residual mercury content decreases with increasing trituration time.

The example given in fig. 54b is a combination of the two graphs given in fig. 54a.

Because the actual form of both fig. 53 and 54 depends strongly upon the choice of the amalgam alloy, the instructions of the manufacturers should be followed precisely. Furthermore, their directions as to the choice of the mixing machine or capsules to be used should be followed as well. For it could happen that one alloy can be triturated in a certain capsule but not in another one.

### 4.4.4. Time between trituration and condensation

The influence of the delay time between trituration and condensation upon the residual mercury content is given in fig. 55.

The influence of the trituration time upon the residual mercury content is given in fig. 54.

The relation between delay time and amount of porosity is represented in fig. 56.

Because more mercury is used between trituration and condensation with increasing delay time, and therefore less mercury can be expressed during condensation, the residual mercury content increases with increasing delay time. At a certain time, the amalgam

Fig. 54 a

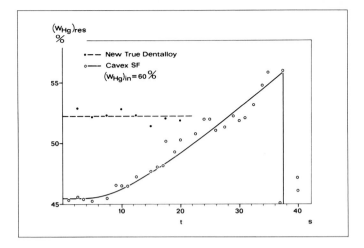

Fig. 54 b

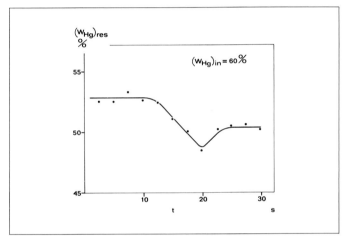

Fig. 54   Dependence of the residual   mercury   content upon the trituration time.

mass cannot be adequately condensed any more because, due to the formation of   reaction   products,   plasticity   decreases. At this time, the (maximum) working time, the residual mercury content increases dramatically. Condensation after this time gives an unacceptable amount of porosity.

## 4.4.5. Condensation

It suffices to say that a carefully controlled condensation process is a prerequisite to get an adequate mercury content as well as a minimum amount of porosity. An increasing condensation pressure gives both less residual mercury (fig. 57) and porosity.

However, for amalgam with a good plasticity, such as most spherical ones, condensation is less critical. In these cases a   high   condensation   pressure   might

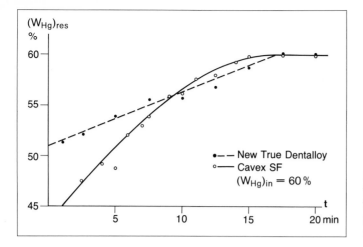

Fig. 55 The influence of the delay time between trituration and condensation upon the residual mercury content.

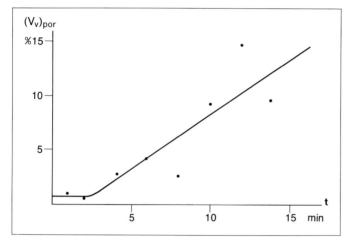

Fig. 56 Dependence of the porosity content upon the delay time between mixing and packing.

jeopardize the quality of the restorations because the amalgam goes up along the packing instrument rather than being adequately condensed. Apart from the condensation pressure, a control of the direction of the condensation thrusts is of ultimate importance. This can be explained on the basis of fig. 58.

In this schematic drawing the direction of the condensation thrust is perpendicular to the floor of the cavity. The arrows refer to the flow of mercury into the direction of the occlusal surface as well as perpendicular to the condensation stroke. As a result, the upper layers of the amalgam restoration as well as parts adjacent to the cavity wall contain more mercury. Generally, the mercury content attains a maximum at the marginal areas of the restoration (see e. g. *Swartz & Phillips,* 1966). A more homogeneously distributed mercury content can be attained by means of condensation which is also directed perpendicular to the cavity walls rather

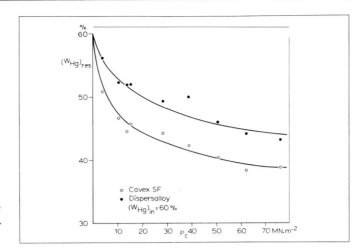

Fig. 57 Residual mercury content as a function of condensation pressure.

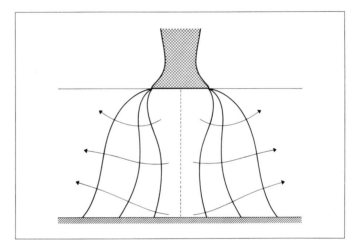

Fig. 58 Distribution of the condensation pressure. Arrows refer to the flow directions of mercury (schematically according to Jørgensen, 1977).

than parallel to them. Extending this concept further, overfilling the cavity gives a better distribution of mercury as well as lower mercury content of the upper layers, especially at the margins of the restorations. Thus the porosity at the margins will be decreased.

### 4.4.6. Carving, burnishing and polishing

Carving, burnishing and polishing influence the structure of the restoration surface substantially. This surface is ex-tremely important because it is the first barrier against corrosive attacks from the oral environment. As found by *Boyer, Edie & Chan* (1977) carving gives a rough surface, whereby deep pores are present at the surface. During both carving and burnishing, the tin compounds are smeared over the surface. After these treatments, the original alloy particles can be hardly detected in the upper layers *(Rupp, Fred & Waterstrat, 1977)*.

Polishing turned out to give the

smoothest surface. It must be stressed here that an increase of polishing does not imply a smoother surface. Because the $\gamma_2$ phase is a relatively soft phase the abrasives remove this phase more easily than the other phases, whereby the $\gamma_2$ phase at the surface might be removed almost completely for long polishing times. As a result, the surface does not shine because of the relatively rough surface. Therefore, the time taken for polishing should not be too long.

## References

Averette, D. F., Hochman, R. F. & Marek, M. (1978): The Effects of Corrosion in Vitro on the Structure and Properties of Dental Amalgam. J. Dent. Res. **57**, Special Issue A, paper 361.

Bergdahl, G. (1973): Residual Mercury and Amalgam Quantity in Conventional and Wet Techniques. Scand. J. Dent. Res. **81**, 260.

Boyer, D. B., Edie, J. W. & Chan, K. C. (1977): Distribution of Phases on Amalgam Surfaces. J. Dent. Res. **56**, Special Issue B, paper 374.

Darvell, B. W. (1976): Strength of Dispersalloy Amalgam. Br. Dent. J. **141**, 273.

Eames, W. B. (1959): Preparation and Condensation of Amalgam with Low Mercury-Alloy Ratio. J. Am. Dent. Assoc. **58**, 78.

Eames, W. B., Tharp, L. G. & Hibbard, E. D. (1973): The Effects of Saliva Contamination on Dental Amalgam. J. Am. Dent. Ass. **86**, 652.

Espevik, S. (1977a): Creep of Dental Amalgam and its Phases. Scand. J. Dent. Res. **85**, 492.

Espevik, S. (1977b): Creep and Phase Transformation in Dental Amalgam. J. Dent. Res. **56**, 36.

Espevik, S. (1977c): Effect of Trituration on Dimensional Changes of Dental Amalgam. Acta Odontol. Scand. **35**, 251.

Hals, E., Nernaes, A., Simonson, T. L., Andreassen, B. H., Bie, T., Halse, A., Das, T. K. & Gjerdet, N. R. (1975): Experimental and Natural Lesions around Silver Amalgam Fillings, in: Proceedings of the International Symposium on Amalgam and Tooth-Coloured Restorative Material. Ed. Van Amerongen, A. J., Dippel, H. W., Spanauf, A. J. & Vrijhoef, M. M. A. Dental School, University of Nijmegen, p. 19.

Holland, G. A. & Asgar, K. (1974): Some Effects on the Phases of Amalgam Induced by Corrosion. J. Dent. Res. **53**, 1245.

Jensen, S. J. (1977): Phase Content of a High Copper Dental Silver Amalgam. Scand. J. Dent. Res. **85**, 297.

Jørgensen, K. D., Esbensen, A. L. & Borring-Møller, G. (1966): The Effect of Porosity and Mercury Content upon the Strength of Silver Amalgam. Acta Odontol. Scand. **5**, 535.

Jørgensen, K. D. (1972): The Strength of Corroded Amalgam. Acta Odontol. Scand. **30**, 33.

Jørgensen, K. D., Christiansen, I. & Esbensen, A. L. (1973): Mercuroscopic Expansion of Dental Amalgams. Tandlaegebladet, **77**, 389.

Jørgensen, K. D. (1975): Evaluation of Amalgam Alloys and Amalgam Properties with Special Reference to Corrosion and Creep of Amalgam, in: Proceedings of the International Symposium on Amalgam and Tooth-Coloured Restorative Material. Ed. Van Amerongen, A. J., Dippel, H. W., Spanauf, A. J. & Vrijhoef, M. M. A. Dental School, University of Nijmegen, p. 9.

Jørgensen, K. D. (1977): Amalgame in der Zahnheilkunde. Carl Hanser, München.

Mahler, D. B. & Mitchem, J. C. (1964): Transverse Strength of Amalgam. J. Dent. Res. **43**, 121.

Mahler, D. B. & Adey, J. E. (1977): Creep versus Microstructure of Amalgam. J. Dent. Res. **56**, Special Issue A, paper 144.

Mahler, D. B., Adey, J. D. & Marantz, R. L. (1978): Evaluation of Three High-Cu Amalgams. J. Dent. Res. **57**, Special Issue A, paper 197.

Malhotra, M. L. & Asgar, K. (1978):
Investigation of Metallurgical Phases in High Copper Amalgams Containing Varying Mercury. J. Dent. Res. **57,** Special Issue A, paper 194.

Marek, M. & Okabe, T. (1977):
Corrosion Behavior of Structural Phases in High Copper Dental Amalgams. J. Dent. Res. **56,** Special Issue A, paper 239.

Mateer, R. S. & Reitz, C. D. (1970):
Corrosion of Amalgam Restorations. J. Dent. Res. **49,** 399.

Nadal, R., Phillips, R. W. & Swartz, M. L. (1961):
Clinical Investigation on the Relation of Mercury to the Amalgam Restoration: II. J. Am. Dent. Assoc. **63,** 488.

Okabe, T., Mitchell, R., Butts, M. B. & Fairhurst, C. W. (1977):
Amalgamation Reaction of Dispersalloy and High Copper Single Composition Alloys. J. Dent. Res. **56,** Special Issue B, paper 378.

Otani, H., Jesser, W. A. & Wilsdorf, H. G. F. (1973):
The In Vivo and In Vitro Corrosion Products of Dental Amalgams. J. Biomed. Mater. Res. **7,** 523.

Rupp, N. W., Fred, S. R. & Waterstrat, R. M. (1977):
The Surface Distribution of Tin-Rich Phases in Dental Amalgams. J. Dent. Res. **56,** Special Issue B, paper 371.

Sarkar, N. K., Marshall, G. W., Moser, J. B. & Greener, E. H. (1975):
In Vivo and In Vitro Corrosion Products of Dental Amalgam. J. Dent. Res. **54,** 1031.

Swartz, M. L. & Phillips, R. W. (1966):
Residual Mercury Content of Amalgam Restorations and its Influence on Compressive Strength. J. Dent. Res. **35,** 458.

Sweeney, A. B. & Burns, C. (1961):
Effect of Mercury-Alloy Ratio on Physical Properties of Amalgams. J. Amer. Dent. Assoc. **63,** 374.

Taylor, D. F. (1972):
Porosity in Silver-Tin Amalgams. J. Biomed. Mater. Res. **6,** 289.

Vrijhoef, M. M. A. & Driessens, F. C. M. (1974a):
Investigation of the Phase Composition of Six Dental Amalgams by X-Ray Diffraction. J. Biomed. Mater. Res. **8,** 443.

Vrijhoef, M. M. A. & Driessens, F. C. M. (1974b):
On the Static Creep of Dental Amalgam. J. Dent. Res. **53,** 1138.

Vrijhoef, M. M. A. & Driessens, F. C. M. (1975a):
Ageing at 37°C versus Creep of Dental Amalgam. J. Dent. Res. **54,** 679.

Vrijhoef, M. M. A. & Driessens, F. C. M. (1975b):
The Primary Factor of the Creep Resistance of Dispersant Amalgams. J. Oral. Rehabil. **2,** 165.

Vrijhoef, M. M. A. & Driessens, F. C. M. (1975c):
Dimensional Change and Creep of Amalgams from (un)annealed Commercial Alloys. J. Dent. Res. **54,** Special Issue A, IADR, paper L168.

Vrijhoef, M. M. A. & Jensen, S. J. (1977):
Chemical Composition, Particle Form and Annealing Temperature of Amalgam Alloy versus Creep of the Resulting Amalgam. J. Bioeng. **1,** 105.

Young, F. A. & Wilsdorf, H. G. F. (1972):
The Effect of Cleaning an Experimental Spherical $Ag_3Sn$ Alloy on the Tensile Strength and Fracture of Dental Amalgam. J. Biomed. Mater. Res. **6,** 81.

# 5. Technical Considerations

## 5.1. Selection of Alloy and Mercury

A great deal of different brands of amalgam alloy are available on the dental market. Before deciding which product to purchase a thorough investigation of the available alloys is essential. Different criteria can be employed to such a selective investigation. The fact whether an alloy is certified according to a dental specification (e. g. ADA or ISO specification) might be used as a first selection criterion. However, selecting from the certified alloys is still a tremendous task. For example, an approximate number of 150 different amalgam alloys are on the certification list of the ADA (conventional composition or high copper; zinc or non-zinc; regular-, fine- or micro-cut; lathe cut, spherical or admixture; slow, regular or fast setting; . . .). In principle, each of these alloys is available in different forms (bulk powder; pellets; pre-capsulated). The individual general practitioner might make a choice from the alternatives on the basis of workability, setting time and other factors. However, in our opinion, the durability of the ultimate restoration should occupy the centre of interest. At present, both marginal fracture and corrosion of amalgam restorations get all the attention. As for the marginal breakdown fig. 40 might be the basis of such a selection of an alloy. However, a warning is necessary here. Fig. 40 was made in spring 1978 and should be considered as a snapshot indication. As time goes by, the existing amalgam alloys are modified and new ones will be introduced. Furthermore, new research reports become available. Therefore it is recommended to screen the literature from time to time. Generally speaking, results of research are reported at an early stage at the annual meeting of the International Association for Dental Research. The Dental Materials Group collects all these papers with regard to dental materials as presented within the respective session of that group. These papers are reproduced on microfilms and are available within a couple of months at a very low price. Although corrosion phenomena such as roughness and discoloration are not completely correlated, as a first approximation, marginal fracture might be taken as an indication of these corrosion characteristics in case of conventional composition amalgams. Unfortunately, only a few data are available with respect to roughness and discoloration. After selecting on the basis of marginal fracture, the general practitioner might make a proper final decision taking into account the workability, setting time and other factors.

First requirement for an adequate condensation of the amalgam is a good plasticity of the amalgam mix. In earlier days pre-amalgamated amalgam alloys were very popular because their plasticity was relatively excellent. However, at present it is not necessary any more to pre-amalgamate the amalgam alloys in order to get a good plasticity of the amalgam mix. By adjusting certain steps of the manufacturing process such as the different heat treatments the manufacturer might obtain an acceptable plasticity as well. Furthermore, the particle form substantially influences the plasticity as well. Only a few years ago the spherical amalgam alloys arose a considerable excitement in the dental profession because of their plasticity. Next to the particle shape, the particle size is important equally. According as the particle size decreases (other factors being kept constant!) the plasticity decreases. We like to stress here that the above mentioned statement holds true for freshly triturated amalgam mixes. In case if the condensation is delayed for five or ten minutes the setting rate should be taken into account. As pointed out in section 3.3.1.1. the different procedures such as condensing, carving and polishing impose upon the amalgam material different requirements. Therefore, if problems with the setting of a specific dental amalgam are encountered it is essential to realize at which particular procedure in the manipulation they arise. Otherwise, confusion of the tongues is inevitable. If the manufacturers introduce a new type of amalgam such a confusion occurs quite frequently. As a result of it, the manufacturers are bombarded with the most inconsistent complaints about the setting rates.

If one group of the dental practitioners advocates the setting rate to be too low, the other group stresses it to be too high. Both groups might be right. This might be explained by means of fig. 59. The setting curve depicted in this graph corresponds with an amalgam which remains plastic during a certain time and, apparently, hardly hardens at the early stages. However, once it starts hardening all proceeds very quickly. Because carving should take place at this stage, time is relatively short to do this. A fast working practitioner will have no problem in the carving phase. However, during condensation, too much of time is available for this operator. Therefore, the fast working practitioner will complain that "the amalgam never gets hard". Another, slow working, dentist will experience no problem at all during condensation. However, for this practitioner too short a time is available for the carving procedure. Contrary to the fast working colleague, this practitioner will complain that the "amalgam sets much too quickly". A type of curve as shown in fig. 59 is frequently observed for the group of amalgams made from spherical alloys.

Section 3.3.2.1. gives a snapshot impression of some commercial amalgams as far as the strength during setting is concerned. It is self-evident that a regular screening of the literature is necessary. It should be stressed here that the maximum time available for condensation and/or carving is very short for some of the new high copper amalgams. Probably this is a resultant of both the demand of the profession for fast(er) setting amalgam systems and the fact that the manufacturers hardly have any experience with these amalgam alloys. It is likely that the inappropriate terminology related to the hardening amalgam plays a role as well. Some of these

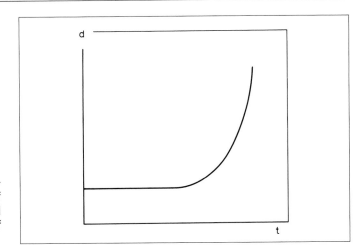

Fig. 59 Schematical representation of the degree of setting (d) of some dental amalgam as a function of time (t).

systems can hardly be manipulated by the average general practitioner, whereas an average student is not able to obtain a reasonable result at all. It is speculated that the characteristics during carving and polishing improve accordingly as particle size decreases. It is reasonable to assume that polishing is easier for the modern non-gamma-2 amalgams (see section 4.4.6). For some amalgams an after-carve burnish might be sufficient whereby a completing polishing session would be superfluous, and therefore could be omitted from the procedure. The reader should follow the developments in this field carefully. Unfortunately, at this time no definite conclusions can be drawn. Although most amalgam alloys do not show up undesirable changes, during storage, there might be some unfavourable changes for a minor part of the commercial alloys. It should be stressed therefore not to purchase large amounts of alloy.

Apart from a careful selection of the amalgam alloy a proper choice of a high quality mercury is of great importance as well. The mercury must be pure (less than 0.02% non volatile residue) whereas surface contaminants must be absent. Purchasing a brand which satisfies the requirements of some dental specification guarantees a sufficient quality and therefore it is a good policy.

## 5.2. Proportioning of Alloy and Mercury

Theoretically, a high initial mercury content might be reduced during condensation so that an acceptable residual mercury content is obtained (relatively high condensation pressure; overfilling). However, in general, residual mercury content increases according as the initial mercury content increases (see fig. 51). Only under very specific conditions the residual mercury content might be independent of the initial mercury content. Generally, the initial mercury content is very important as any deviation from the recommended alloy/mercury ratio may be detrimen-

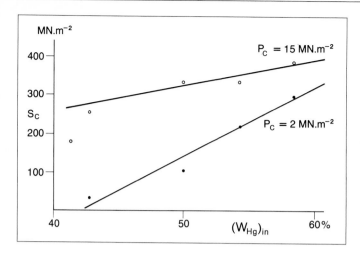

Fig. 60 The influence of the initial mercury content upon the compressive strength of Standalloy F. The respective condensation pressures are 2 MN/m² and 15 MN/m² (data according to Dermann, 1978).

tal to the properties of the amalgam. A relatively high initial mercury percentage is detrimental unless sufficient mercury or the overfilled portions are removed during condensation (see fig. 45). On the other hand, a relatively low initial mercury content might jeopardize the properties as well. For example fig. 60 illustrates that the compressive strength of some commercial amalgam is much more dependent upon the condensation pressure for a low initial mercury content than for a high initial mercury percentage. From fig. 60 it might be deduced that a too dry mix has much more negative effect upon the compressive strength than a too wet one. In general, it might be stated as well that the risks of a too wet mix are smaller than those of a too dry one. Because both a too dry mix and a too wet amalgam involve negative effects a careful proportioning of alloy and mercury should be carried out.

The most convenient way of proportioning for a general practitioner is selecting a precapsulated amalgam system (see fig. 61). In this case the manufacturer is responsible for an accurate proportioning of both amalgam alloy and mercury. *Eames, Mack & Auvenshire* (1970) published data as to the accuracy of precapsulated systems. Some of them showed up unacceptable variations with respect to the initial mercury content. Unfortunately, no recent data are available. In the near future demands as to the accuracy of predosed amalgam alloy and mercury will be included in the specifications so that selection of a certified precapsulated system is a safe policy which guarantees a sufficient accuracy of the initial mercury content. The amalgam alloy might be purchased as pellets as well. In this case, the chair assistant must take care of an accurate proportioning of the mercury (see fig. 62). If the conditions are optimal most mercury dispensers will be reliable. The mercury should be clean so as to guarantee an accurate dosage. The dispenser should be filled for at least 1/4. During dosing the dispenser bottle should be kept in a vertical position. Most mercury dispensers can be tilted to an angle of 22° without any major

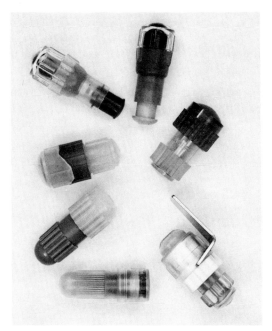

Fig. 61 a

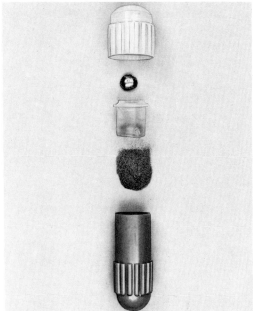

Fig. 61 b

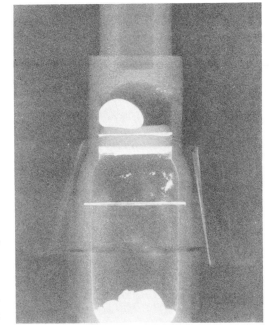

Fig. 61 a    Some commercial precapsulated systems.

Fig. 61 b    Exploded capsule.

Fig. 61 c    X-ray picture of a commercial precapsulated system showing the different compartments of alloy and mercury (Courtesy of Dr. W. H. J. M. van Immerseel).

Fig. 61 c

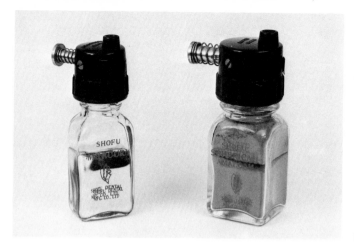

Fig. 62 A commercial mercury and alloy dispenser.

errors. However, tipping to an angle of 45° gives a substantial error which might result in an unacceptable amalgam mix and thereby jeopardize the properties of the amalgam restoration (Eames et al., 1970). Of course, proportioning alloy powder by means of a powder dispenser is possible as well (see fig. 62). In this case adjustment of the dispenser as well as manipulation during dispensing are very critical. A frequently repeated check on the adjustment is necessary. Standardized shaking of the bottle and tapping it on the table before dispensing are required. This is necessary in order to omit segregation of the alloy powder and to guarentee a constant particle size distribution as well as a constant weight from mix to mix. It is clear that both the alloy powder and mercury can be weighed by means of some type of a balance. Because of its cumbersomeness this proportioning procedure has gone out of use almost completely. At last some attention must be given to the nomenclature related to the initial mercury content. It is common practice amongst manufacturers to refer to

either the so-called mercury/alloy ratio or to the alloy/mercury ratio. Moreover, manufacturers refer to the initial mercury content in terms of the weight percentage of the mercury. The relation between the mercury/alloy ratio and the initial weight percentage of mercury is depicted in fig. 63.

## 5.3. Trituration

The objective of the trituration is a complete wetting of the amalgam alloy particles with mercury. Apart from factors related to the manufacturing process such as chemical composition and heat treatments the presence of an oxide layer, covering the alloy particles more or less completely, plays an important role. Removing the oxide layer is one of the major objectives during the early stages of mixing. The mechanical violence during the trituration process makes it possible to break up the oxide layer, which will enable the mercury to wet the alloy particles. The oldest form

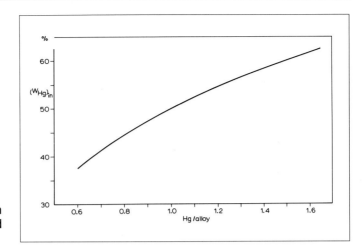

Fig. 63 Relation between initial mercury/alloy ratio and initial mercury content.

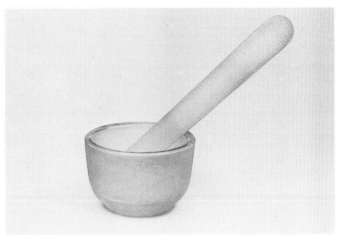

Fig. 64 Mortar and pestle for hand trituration.

of mixing is carried out by means of a mortar and a pestle (fig. 64). An adequate training and minimization of the variations during hand mixing are conditions to obtain an optimal amalgam mix. Therefore, factors such as pressure exerted on the mix, number of revolutions per minute, inclination of the pestle relative to the mortar, surface roughness of both mortar and pestle, and other factors should be carefully controlled. Although really very good, results might be obtained (see fig. 27)

hand mixing is almost not practiced any more. A standardized amalgam mass of adequate quality can be obtained much easier and in a shorter time by means of a mechanical amalgamator (fig. 65). Mechanical trituration eliminates several sources of variation of the hand mixing process. Furthermore it is advantageous initially to use less mercury to obtain a satisfactory amalgam mass. The effectivity of the amalgamator depends on factors such as size and form of the capsule, geometry and

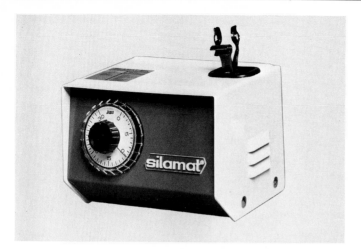

Fig. 65 a

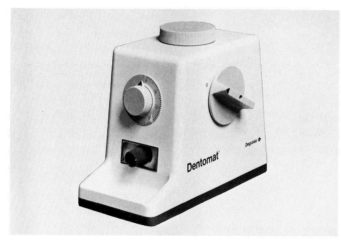

Fig. 65 b

Fig. 65 Two mechanical amalgamators.

(a) Silamat machine.

(b) Dentomat. This machine is very popular because both proportioning and mixing can be done with it.

distance of the thrust as well as the number of revolutions per minute.

*Lautenschlager, Rechtien & Norling* (1972) reported that the (theoretical) optimum capsule length occurs if the ratio of the capsule length to the travel distance is 1.6 approximately. Viscous drag between capsule and amalgam mix is expected to make this ratio slightly lower. It should be noted that the frequency of the amalgamator per se does not influence the optimum ratio of the capsule length to thrust distance. As a matter of fact an increasing frequency creates more impacts per second at a higher level of violence. This might explain the fact that, in general, high speed amalgamators need no pestle in the capsule while the choice of a low speed necessitates the use of a pestle. Because mechanical trituration depends upon several factors, the instructions of the manufacturer of the amalgam alloy should be followed strictly as to recommendations with regard to variables such as the mechanical mixing device,

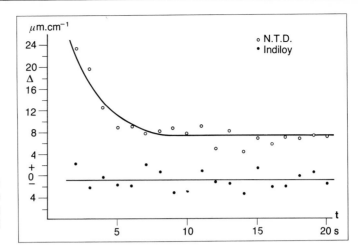

Fig. 66 The influence of the trituration time upon the dimensional change during hardening of two commercial amalgams.

the use of a pestle and the mixing time. For an evaluation of several amalgamators it is referred to a publication by *Eames* (1972) written for the Council on Dental Materials and Devices. Once the amalgamator, capsule and pestle have been chosen, major errors can be related to the trituration time. Some typical cases of the influence of the trituration time upon dimensional change during hardening, compressive strength and creep are given in the figures 66 to 68.

It is generally accepted that the dimensional change decreases as the trituration time increases. However, dimensional change of most of the present-day amalgams is rather independent of the trituration time over a wide range. For relatively short trituration times commercial amalgams show up the generally accepted dependence of dimensional change upon trituration time (e. g. the upper curve in fig. 66). For several amalgams this stage cannot be determined experimentally because of the bad plasticity of the amalgam mix. For relatively short mixing times compressive strength increases according as trituration time increases (e. g. the lower curve in fig. 67). Then it is rather independent of the mixing time over a wide range. For very long trituration time, the strength is expected to decrease with increasing mixing time. *Osborne* et al. (1977) have reported a single case. In general, such long times are not realistic because of the resulting poor plasticity of the amalgam mass at these mixing times.

Two examples of the influence of the trituration time upon the creep are given in fig. 68. For one amalgam the creep is independent of the trituration time over a wide range. In another case creep increases with increasing mixing time. For relatively short trituration times *Osborne* et al. (1977) reported creep to decrease with increasing mixing time (see fig. 36) till a minimum creep value is attained. However afterwards this minimum creep would increase again with increasing mixing time. For major part of the present-day amalgams such a minimum is not realistic. A minor part might show up such a minimum.

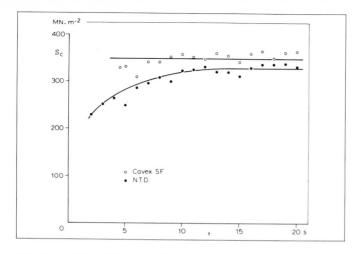

Fig. 67 The influence of the trituration time upon the compressive strength after hardening of two commercial amalgams.

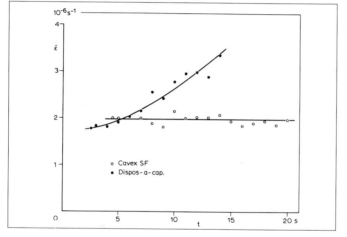

Fig. 68 The influence of the trituration time upon the creep of two commercial amalgams.

From the figures 66 to 68 it might be concluded that both undertrituration and overtrituration might jeopardize the properties of the amalgam and thereby the functioning of the resulting restoration under oral conditions. Therefore, an accurate adjustment of the mixing time is very important. It is generally accepted that the consequences of an overtrituration are less than those of an undertrituration. However, both jeopardize the quality and stability of the amalgam restoration.

The probability of a bad amalgam mix is minimized if the dental team is keen on doing a good job and therefore pays a lot of attention to the trituration. The first indications whether the amalgam mix is good can be already observed during the mixing process itself. During trituration a sound change takes place. This sound change is an indication that the amalgam alloy and mercury have been throughly mixed and that a globule has been created. After mixing there are several simple expedients to judge the

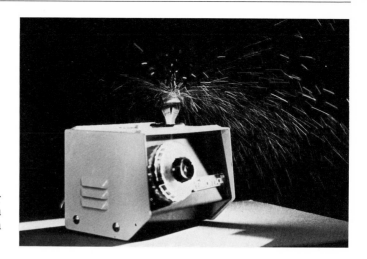

Fig. 69 Spray of tiny mercury drops escaping from a
capsule during trituration (a
simulated picture).

quality of the amalgam mix *(Eames,*
*1976).* The amalgam mix should be
smooth and coherent. If it is gently
pressed between the fingers the imprint
of the fingers should be reproduced,
whereby a slight amount of mercury
should appear on the surface. This
minimal amount of mercury pressed
out of the amalgam mix is a condition for
a good adaptability as well as to make it
possible to prevent lamination during
condensation. An undertriturated mass
shows up a more or less granular tex-
ture and will be experienced as less
coherent during condensation. The ex-
cessively overtriturated amalgam becomes much more noisy during packing,
which is due to the fact that the formation of the matrix phases is already
far advanced. The overtriturated amalgam sets too rapidly for an adequate
condensation and carving.

Apart from optimizing the properties of
the amalgam restoration with an adequate control of the trituration, the dental team should be aware of the fact that
the mixing process involves dangers as
to the health. Especially in case of high
speed amalgamators, a spray of tiny
drops might escape from the capsule
*(Nixon & Rowbotham,* 1971; fig. 69).
The non-disposable capsules should
be cleaned thoroughly at the critical places. Non-disposables capsules
should not be used more than 30—50
times *(Lugassy & Kupps,* 1978). Unfortunately, not all disposable capsules are
safe as far as mercury leakage is concerned *(Castagnola & Wirz,* 1973). Once
a disposable capsule is opened it should
not be used any more. At present a lot of
changes are occurring in the field of disposable capsules. Therefore, a regular
screening of the literature is necessary.

## 5.4. Condensation

After the amalgam mass has been
made, it should be packed into the prepared cavity as quickly as possible because the setting reactions already are
proceeding whereby new matrix phases

are being formed. During condensation, these already formed crystals of the matrix phases might be broken up and weaken the matrix. Furthermore, plasticity of the amalgam mass will become inferior. Therefore properties such as the strength, creep and corrosion resistance will deteriorate with increasing delay time between mixing and packing. For two different amalgams, the influence of the delay time between mixing and packing upon compressive strength after hardening is given in fig. 70. From this graph it is obvious that the influence upon the compressive strength of a slow setting amalgam is much less than in case of a fast setting system. This is quite understandable on the basis of the formation rate of the matrix phases. For a regular setting system the maximum allowable delay time after trituration varies from 3—4 minutes approximately. In case of some fast setting systems the mix already should be discarded after 1—2 minutes. Therefore, for a large restoration several mixes may be necessary.

The aim of condensation is to force the amalgam into the cavity in such a way that it adapts itself to the remaining tooth structures as close as possible. The amount of porosity should be as low as possible whereas no lamination between the different mixes inserted into the cavity should occur. During condensation, the dentist should aim at this situation as much as possible. Therefore, the operator should be aware of the fact that the occurrence of voids is greatest in the bottom corners (Silness & Hegdahl, 1970). The mercury content increases from the floor of the cavity to the occlusal surface, whereas the mercury content of the margins is higher than in the central parts of the res-

toration. Generally, the mercury content attains a maximum at the marginal area of the restoration (Swartz & Phillips, 1966). Depending on the condensation technic as well as on the amalgam alloy used, the mercury content might show up variations of several weight percentages (see e. g. Wilson, Phillips & Norman, 1957; Swartz & Phillips, 1966; Bergdahl, 1973). Unacceptable mercury content variations due to a lack of proper condensation and overfilling might be as great as 15 wt.% (Flögel, 1964). Although there are many different condensation technics it is unlikely that the differences between carefully carried out technics are of any importance. This indication might be deduced from both laboratory results (cf. chapter 3) and initial clinical investigations (Letzel et al., 1978). The greatest risk during condensation occurs if the mix is undertriturated, too dry, big amalgam increments rather than if small ones are used, or in the case that setting is already advanced too much. In these cases voids will occur in the amalgam, no optimal adaptation to the cavity wall will be obtained whereas lamination will be present because subsequent amalgam increments will not be sufficiently bonded together. As already explained in section 4.4.5. a more homogeneously distributed mercury content can be attained by means of condensation which is also directed as much as possible perpendicular to the cavity walls rather than parallel to them. Furthermore, overfilling the cavity gives a better distribution of mercury as well as a lower mercury content of the upper layer; especially at the margins of the restoration.

The oldest form of condensation is carried out by hand (fig. 71). Although

100

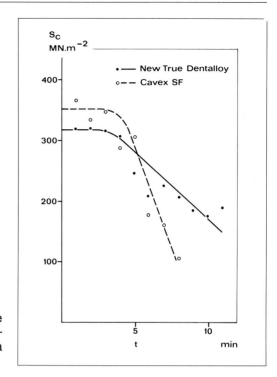

Fig. 70 The influence of the delay time between mixing and packing upon the compressive strength after hardening for a regular setting and a fast setting amalgam.

this form probably is still common practice, mechanical condensation (fig. 72) becomes more and more popular, because of its ergonometric advantages such as less fatigue and a shorter condensation time. Once the dentist has made his choice for either mechanical or hand condensation, the proper choice of the size of the condensation point is of ultimate importance. For a given condensation force, the area of the condensation point determines the pressure exerted by the dentist. The relation between condensation pressure and area of the packing plugger is given in fig. 73. The condensation force was assumed to be 10N (1 kgf approximately). A condensation pressure corresponding with a force of x N ($\cong$ x/10 kgf) might be obtained from fig.

73 by multiplication with a constant x/10.

At present, there is no agreement about the value necessary for an optimal condensation procedure. One of the reasons is that the optimal condensation pressure differs from alloy to alloy. For instance, an amalgam from a spherical alloy necessitates a lower condensation pressure than one from a lathe cut alloy.

From literature it is clear that during the last 50 years the packing pressures have substantially decreased. In the first decades of this century, packing pressures in the order of 56 $MN/m^2$, although not common practice, were not unusual (see e. g. *Ward & Scott,* 1932); especially by practitioners doing a lot of gold foil work. If one uses a 2 mm condensation

Table 6
The condensation force (in N; division by 10 gives kgf approximately) for some selected condensation pressures found in literature as a function of the diameter of a cilindrical condensation plugger.

| Condensation pressure (MN/m²) | Diameter of Cilindrical Condenser (mm) | | | | | |
|---|---|---|---|---|---|---|
| | 0.8 | 1.0 | 1.5 | 1.75 | 2.0 | 2.5 |
| 56 | 28 | 44 | 99 | 135 | 176 | 275 |
| 14 | 7.0 | 11 | 25 | 34 | 44 | 69 |
| 9.0 | 4.5 | 7.1 | 16 | 22 | 28 | 44 |
| 5.3 | 2.7 | 4.2 | 9.4 | 13 | 17 | 26 |
| 2.5 | 1.3 | 2.0 | 4.4 | 6.0 | 7.8 | 12 |
| 2.0 | 1.0 | 1.6 | 3.5 | 4.8 | 6.3 | 9.8 |

instrument this necessitates a condensation force of 180 N ($\cong$ 18 kgf) approximately, which is very difficult to attain.

With a 1.5 mm point such a pressure requires a force of 100 N approximately (see table 6), whereas a small 0.8 condenser still requires a force of 30 N ($\cong$ 3 kgf) approximately. In those days, it was common practice to remind the dental students that an amalgam restoration was not adequately condensed if the arm of the operator did not feel tired after the restorative procedure. Still *Markley* (1951) stated that "it is likely that if the operator's arm does not ache after condensing a large filling, the filling is not well condensed". More recently, lower condensation pressures have been reported. *Peyton* et al. (1968) state that the pressure used by most of the clinicians is about 140 kgf/cm² ($\cong$ 14 MN/m²). As far as amalgams from conventional lathe cut alloys are concerned *Nagai* et al. (1971) give a value of 53 kgf/cm² ($\cong$ 5.3 MN/m²), whereas *Forsten* (1971) considers a value of 90 kgf/cm² ($\cong$ 9 MN/m²) to be sufficient. *Forsten* (1971) gives a condensation

pressure of 20 kgf/cm² ($\cong$ 2 MN/m²) for amalgams from spherical amalgam alloys, whereas *Nagai* et al. (1971) give a value of 25 kgf/cm² ($\cong$ 2.5 MN/m²). From table 6 it is obvious that a condensation pressure of 2 MN/m² for an amalgam from a spherical alloy is attained very easily; a small 0.8 mm condenser point requires only 1 N ($\cong$ 0.1 kgf) whereas a big 2.5 mm condenser needs 10 N ($\cong$ 1 kgf). Because condensation forces have been reduced a factor 10—30 in a relatively short time, it is understandable that several dentists had quite a lot of trouble when trying spherical amalgam alloys at their introduction 10 years ago. If a 50—100 N (5—10 kgf) condensation force is applied to the amalgam from a spherical alloy the amalgam "is launched from the cavity and will hit the ceiling" rather than being condensed in the cavity.

Ergonometrically it is not clear which condensation forces are favourable. According to *Skinner & Phillips* (1960) for working under oral conditions 4.5 kgf ($\cong$ 45 N) is a maximum the clinician might apply. *Mahler & Mitchem* (1965) reported an average force of 1.4—1.8 kgf

Fig. 71 a

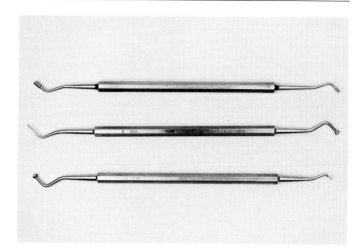

Fig. 71 b

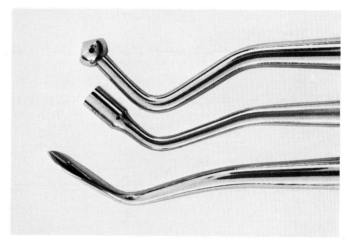

Fig. 71 a and b  Some hand pluggers, burnishing and carving instruments.

($\cong$ 14–18 N). *Moffa & Jenkins* (1971) reported 0.5–1.5 kgf ($\cong$ 5–15 N), whereas *Basker & Wilson* (1968) stated the average condensation force to be 1.3 kgf ($\cong$ 13 N).

It is feasible that major part of the lathe cut and admixture type alloys can be adequately condensed with a pressure of 53 kgf/cm$^2$ ($\cong$ 5.3 MN/m$_2$), which can be easily attained by means of a 2 mm condenser. Table 6 might help to select a proper condenser size. It is strongly advised to use a small conden-ser (e. g. 0.8 mm) at the initial stages of condensing in order to pack into retentive grooves and cavo-surface margins. Medium-sized condensers should be used to pack the bulk of the restoration, whereas the large instruments only should be used for the last portions of the occlusal surface. From table 6 it is clear that the term "small", "medium" and "large" are very relative and that the actual condenser size depends on the amalgam alloy (and cavity preparation!). Apart from the con-

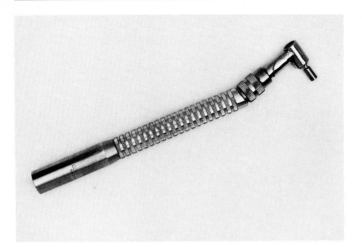

Fig. 72a

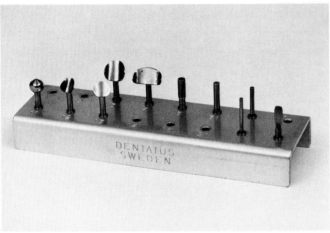

Fig. 72b

Fig. 72 A mechanical packing instrument (a) and its accessories (b).

denser size and packing force, the surface condition of the condensation instrument is important as well. Smooth condensers tend to slide across the amalgam whereas the serrated condenser has more grip on the amalgam mass. A disadvantage of the serrated condenser points is that they are relatively difficult to clean so that they easily clog and get contaminated. At last, it should be stressed here that the condensation time plays an important role as well. A twenty thrusts for each portion is recommended. Care should be taken not to exceed the maximum condensation time available.

The use of a mechanical packing instrument allows the practitioner to conserve his energy. However, an initial clinical study (*Letzel* et al., 1978) shows that the quality and stability of restorations being hand condensed is the same approximately in comparison with restorations condensed with a mechanical packing device. *Eames* et al. (1977) have evaluated major part of the

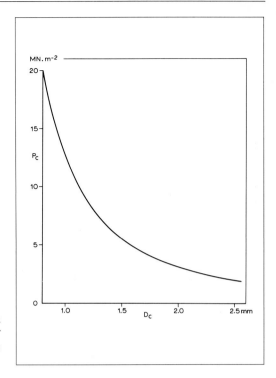

Fig. 73 The condensation pressure $P_c$ as a function of the diameter $D_c$ of a circular packing plugger. The condensation force was assumed to be 10 N ($\cong$ 1 kgf).

available mechanical condensers. For the technical descriptions and the abilities of the respective condensers the reader is referred to this work.

## 5.5. Carving, Burnishing and Polishing

After condensation, the restoration is carved in order to reproduce the proper tooth anatomy. Occlusal overhang should be avoided (see fig. 41) because amalgam should be considered as a brittle material. Small isolated parts of amalgam in the marginal area due to extremely deep carving should be avoided as well. Apart from structural weakness deep pits and fissures are prone to

corrosive attacks from the oral environment. The amalgam is ready for carving if it is sufficiently hardened. If carving is started too early, the amalgam is so plastic that it is pulled out from the tooth structure.

After carving, the restoration should be given either an additional burnishing or polishing treatment so that a smooth surface is obtained. The first clinical investigation as to this point done by *Leinfelder* et al. (1977) showed controversial data. For a relatively quickly setting amalgam they reported that post-carve burnishing resulted in less marginal fracture whereby marginal fracture was not affected in case if the restoration was additionally polished. However, *Leinfelder* et al. (1977) described a negative influence of burnish-

105

ing upon marginal deterioration for a slow setting amalgam. Also in this case polishing of amalgam restorations which had been previously burnished did not improve the situation as to the marginal integrity. In all cases amalgam restorations which were not burnished, showed up less marginal fracture if the restoration was polished. Because of these controversial data it is strongly advised, until more research is done, to be very careful as to the burnishing treatment. As yet, the form of old recommended polishing technic after one or two days should be preferred.

Heat generation should be avoided during polishing. Therefore, polishing under wet conditions is necessary. It must be pointed out here that an increase of the polishing time does not imply a smooth surface. Because the $\gamma_2$ phase is a relatively soft phase, the abrasives remove this phase more easily than the other phases, whereby the $\gamma_2$ phase particles at the surface might be removed almost completely for long polishing times. As a result, the surface does not shine, because of the relatively rough surface. Because of the absence of $\gamma_2$ phase it is expected that polishing is easier for the modern non-$\gamma_2$ amalgams.

## 5.6. Repair of Amalgam Restorations

A failing amalgam restoration should be repaired rather than replaced. New amalgam is condensed to the already present material. It is obvious that the bond between old and new amalgam is the main source of structural weakness of the repaired restoration. Factors such as contamination with saliva and oxidi-

zation of the fractured surface of the old amalgam restoration prevent an effective bond between old and new amalgam (Consani, Ruhnke & Stolf, 1977). Under laboratory conditions, Jørgensen & Saito (1968) were able to obtain a substantially improved bond. Their technic assumes rubbing the surface of the old amalgam with the condenser point in the presence of mercury. Because no oxidization and/or contamination should be present it is not clear whether their technic is a reliable one to be done under oral conditions. Unfortunately, no clinical research is available. Therefore, for the time being this technic should be done in low stress areas.

### References

*Basker, R. M. & Wilson, H. J.* (1968):
Condensation of Amalgam. The Clinical Measurement of Forces and Rates of Packing. Br. Dent. J. **124,** 451.

*Bergdahl, G.* (1973):
Residual Mercury and Amalgam Quantity in Conventional and Wet Techniques. Scand. J. Dent. Res. **81,** 260.

*Castagnola, L. & Wirz, J.* (1973):
Die Quecksilberverdampfung bei der Verarbeitung von Silberamalgam. Schweiz. Mschr. Zahnheilk. **83,** 922.

*Consani, S., Ruhnke, L. A. & Stolf, W. L.* (1977):
Infiltration of a Radioactive Solution into Joined Silver-Amalgam. J. Prosthet. Dent. **37,** 158.

*Dermann, K.* (1978):
Druckfestigkeit von Amalgam in Abhängigkeit vom Stopfdruck und vom Legierungs-Quecksilber-Verhältnis. Dtsch. Zahnärztl. Z. **33,** 480.

*Eames, W. B., Mack, R. M. & Auvenshire, R. C.* (1970):
Accuracy of Mercury/Alloy Proportioning Systems. J. Am. Dent. Assoc. **81,** 137.

Eames, W. B.
(written for the Council on Dental Materials and Devices) (1972):
Status Report on Amalgamators and Mercury/Alloy Proportioners and Disposable Capsules. J. Am. Dent. Assoc. **85,** 928.

Eames, W. B. (1976):
A Clinical View of Dental Amalgam. Dent. Clin. North. Am. **20,** 385.

Eames, W. B., Palmertree, C. O., Zimmermann, L. N. & McNamara, J. F. (1977):
Mechanical Amalgam Condensers Compared. Oper. Dent. **2,** 72.

Flögel, G. E. (1964):
De Invloed van de Condensatiemethode op de Verdeling van Kwik in Amalgaamrestauraties. Ned. Tijdschr. Tandheelk. **71,** 749.

Forsten, L. (1971):
Influence of Manipulation Technique on Early Strength of Different Amalgams. Suom. Hammaslääk. Toim. **67,** 211.

Jørgensen, K. D. & Saito, T. (1968):
Bond Strength of Repaired Amalgam. Acta Odontol. Scand. **26,** 605.

Lautenschlager, E. P., Rechtien, J. J. & Norling, B. K. (1972):
Optimum Trituration Capsule Length. J. Dent. Res. **51,** 1658.

Leinfelder, K. F., Sluder, T. B., Strickland, W. D. & Taylor, D. F. (1977):
Two Year Clinical Evaluation of Burnished Amalgam Restorations. J. Dent. Res. **56,** Special Issue B, paper 251.

Letzel, H., Aardening, Ch. J. M. W., Fick, J. M., Van Leusen, J. & Vrijhoef, M. M. A. (1978):
Condensation Technic versus Clinical Behaviour of Amalgam Restorations. J. Dent. Res. **57,** Special Issue A, paper 497.

Lugassy, A. A. & Kupps, B. (1978):
Amalgam Contamination in Reusable and Double Seal Capsules. J. Dent. Res. **57,** Special Issue A, paper 362.

Mahler, D. B. & Mitchem, J. C. (1965):
Effect of Precondensation Mercury Content on the Physical Properties of Amalgam. J. Am. Dent. Assoc. **71,** 593; reference to unpublished data.

Markeley, M. R. (1951):
Restorations of Silver Amalgam. J. Am. Dent. Assoc. **43,** 133.

Moffa, J. P. & Jenkins, W. A. (1971):
Clinical Evaluation of Amalgam Condensation, IADR Program and Abstracts, paper 739.

Nagai, K., Ohashi, M., Habu, H., Nomoto, K., Nagata, Y., Seto, K. & Arai, F. (1971):
A Study on the Condensation Pressure for Spherical Amalgam. J. Nihon Univ. Sch. Dent. **13,** 133.

Nixon, G. S. & Rowbotham, T. C. (1971):
Mercury Hazards Associated with High Speed Mechanical Amalgamators. Br. Dent. J. **131,** 308.

Osborne, J. W., Phillips, R. W., Norman, R. D., & Swartz, M. L. (1977):
Influence of Certain Manipulative Variables on the Static Creep of Amalgam. J. Dent, Res. **56,** 616.

Peyton, F. A., Asgar, K., Charbeneau, G. T., Craig, R. G. & Myers, G. E. (1968):
Restorative Dental Materials. C. V. Mosby, Saint Louis.

Silness, J. & Hegdahl, T. (1970):
Distribution of Porosity in Spherical Amalgam. Scand. J. Dent. Res. **78,** 69.

Skinner, E. W. & Phillips, R. W. (1960):
The Science of Dental Materials. Saunders, Philadelphia.

Swartz, M. L. & Phillips, R. W. (1966):
Residual Mercury Content of Amalgam Restorations and its Influence on Compressive Strength. J. Dent. Res. **35,** 458.

Ward, M. L. & Scott, E. P. (1932):
Effects of Variations in Manipulation on Dimensional Changes, Crushing Strength and Flow of Amalgams. J. Am. Dent. Assoc. **19,** 1683.

Wilson, R. T., Phillips, R. W. & Norman, R. D. (1957):
Influence of Certain Condensation Procedures upon the Mercury Content of Amalgam Restorations. J. Dent. Res. **36,** 458.

# Index

quintessence
books

Dean L. Johnson/Russell J. Stratton

# Fundamentals of Removable Prosthodontics

Many contemporary clinicians and teachers have training that emphasized the mechanical and laboratory aspects of prosthodontics. Today's educational philosophies stress the relationship of the basic sciences and clinical procedures. It is this concept that led to the writing of "Fundamentals of Removable Prosthodontics." "Fundamentals of Removable Prosthodontics" focuses on the basic knowledge and skills which the general practitioner needs so that he can provide the prosthodontic services required by the majority of his patients. Sophisticated techniques appropriate for graduate or specialty education have been deliberately omitted. As the main thrust of the book centers on information related to patient care, detailed instructions for all laboratory procedures are not included. The clinician who understands the biologic nature of the oral cavity and the physical characteristics of the materials employed will be capable of requesting and evaluating appropriate laboratory services. Perhaps you will find this approach of value in your teaching program.

About 500 pages, 458 illustrations, 17.5 x 24.5 cm, linen bound with gold stamping and dust jacket, price $46, plus handling and 6% sales tax in Illinois.

quintessence
books

Freedman

# Management of the Geriatric Dental Patient

People are living longer; this is inevitably reflected in the composition of the dental practice population. Senior citizens have some oral health problems similar to those of the general population, and other problems that reflect their age and their general health status.

The dentist sees such patients in several settings: his office, homes for the elderly, and—occasionally—in the patient's own home. Each of the settings requires some adaptation if the older patient is to receive care under optimal conditions.

Management of the older patient requires some adjustment on the part of the dentist as well. He must be particularly careful to recognize dental problems associated with long-term use of certain drugs, and he must learn to understand that older patients require special attention. This book will help the concerned dentist to provide optimal care to a growing segment of the population, with minimal disruption of his normal routines.

148 pages, 80 illustrations (59 multi-colored),
17.5 x 24.5 cm, linen bound with gold stamping and dust jacket, price $42, plus handling and 6% sales tax in Illinois.